A Path Less Conventional

A Path Less Conventional

Michael E Morrison

ATHENA PRESS
LONDON

ISBN: 978 1 84748 380 5

First published 2008 by
ATHENA PRESS
Queen's House, 2 Holly Road
Twickenham TW1 4EG
United Kingdom

Extract from *Living Energies: An Exposition of Concepts Related to the Theories of Viktor Schauberger* by Callum Coats, originally published by Gill & MacMillan, reprinted with permission of the author and publisher.

Extract from *Love, Medicine and Miracles* by Bernie S Siegel, published by Rider, reprinted by permission of The Random House Group Ltd.

Extract from *Eternal Echoes* by John O'Donohue, published by Bantam Press, reprinted by permission of The Random House Group Ltd.

Extract from *Asthma Free Naturally: Everything You Need to Know About Taking Control of Your Asthma* by Patrick G McKeown, published by Harper Thorsons, reprinted with kind permission of the author.

Extract from *Breathing* by Michael Sky, Rochester, VT 05767 Copyright © 1990 Inner Traditions/Bear & Co. www.BearandCompanyBooks.com reprinted by permission of the publisher.

Extract from *Vibrational Medicine* by Richard Gerber, Rochester, VT 05767 Copyright © 2001 Inner Traditions/Bear & Co. www.BearandCompanyBooks.com reprinted by permission of the publisher.

Printed for Athena Press

ACKNOWLEDGEMENTS

I would like to thank many who have inspired, perspired and never tired in helping to make this a reality.

Special thanks goes to my parents, Breda and Ed Morrison. Thank you for your support and joie de vivre attitude to life. It opened countless windows of opportunity, allowing me to find my own path.

Thanks to Tony Clarkson for your genial generosity and guidance. I look forward to our time in Brazil together every year. The countless conversations we've had over the last few years have inspired this book.

Thanks to David Begley for allowing use of his work for the cover.

Thanks also to Athena Press for your kind words on receiving and accepting my text. You helped me realise a life goal and I will always thank you for that.

Michael E Morrison

AUTHOR'S NOTE

I was born with cystic fibrosis and lost my younger brother, Ted, to this life-threatening genetic condition. For most families, this would mean tragedy and suffering, painfully retreating from the world at the unfair loss of a child and the suffering of another. However, my mother and father let me be free to embrace the wonder of life, saving me from the restraints of a cotton-wool existence.

The medical profession told them that I would be lucky to see my twelfth birthday. Yet, as I write this, I have celebrated my thirtieth birthday and plan to celebrate many more. My parents' approach has allowed me to lead a life full of opportunity, allowing me to become more than my illness, and this is a wonderful gift.

As I have undergone research over the years, I have come to realise that conventional Western medicine follows a chemical approach to healing that is not always effective. In searching for alternatives, I have come to view my disease differently and discover simple, natural ways that we can trigger healing within ourselves. If you want to heal yourself, as Edward Bach espoused, you must 'tap into the hidden physician within'. Exploring this healer requires you to unmask all and face yourself.

Over the last few years, I have been piecing together a complementary guide to my healing. It has been an empowering exercise, using my body as a human guinea pig, with fantastic results being attained. I have spent my time reading and attending courses and workshops on alternative therapies and on using the body's own power to heal itself. This book describes the range of treatments that can be synergistically employed to bring vitality and well-being.

Although these techniques have been written about and much discussed in other books, their employment for treating a chronic, life-threatening ailment like cystic fibrosis, largely free of conventional means, is unusual. I have been on only a minimal dosage of antibiotics since July 2003 and from being on home intravenous treatment twice a year, I have not had one for several years. I have also reduced my nebuliser count from five a day, back in the summer of 2003, to two a day at present, and I no longer require the use of inhalers. The Cystic Fibrosis Association of Ireland now put my number out to other families across Ireland to inform them about the avenues I have undertaken and some are following my route.

In *A Path Less Conventional*, I aim to give others with ailments, whether it is CF or any other chronic disease, hope that there are ways and means to treat the problem other than those promoted by Western medicine. I have had my ups and downs, but the decision has been mine and I hope that others reading this will learn to take control of their health and steer their way towards healing.

Michael E Morrison

CONTENTS

THE MIRACLE MAN
João de Deus

For those who believe, no words are necessary; for those who do not believe, no words are possible.

Dom Inácio de Loyola

Medicine today is not about cure; it is a band-aid approach to healing – chemically treating the body with antibiotics and following the Newtonian pharmacokinetic (and surgical) approach to healing.

> Disease will never be cured or eradicated by present materialistic methods, for the simple reason that disease in its origin is not material. What we know as disease is an ultimate result produced in the body, the end product of deep and longing forces, and even if material treatment alone is apparently successful this is nothing more than a temporary relief unless the real cause is removed. The modern trend of medical science, by misinterpreting the true nature of disease and concentrating it in materialistic terms in the physical body, has enormously increased its power, firstly by distracting the thoughts of people from its true origin and hence from the effective method of attack, and secondly by localising it in the body, thus obscuring true hope of recovery and raising a mighty disease complex of fear, which should never have existed.[1]

I think that as so many of us don't want a cure, relief is the menu of choice – for to face a cure means to face yourself. Too often, the constant state of activity of our daily lives and the cacophony of noise deafens our ability to see ourselves or be ourselves. Relief, on the other hand, means continuously bypassing the

---

[1] Dr Edward Bach, *Heal Thyself: An Explanation of the Real Cause and Cure of Disease*, Random House UK, newly ed. edition, 2004, p.2

problem and numbing ourselves, allowing our hectic, manic-paced lives to continue under the veil of well-being. When we are in a good, healthy state in our world, we never notice how well we are. Only when illness comes does it shake us to the core and challenge everything about us. In my case, illness took centre stage for the summer of 2003. It unmasked everything and exposed me to the elements of Western healing. I missed out on everything that summer – work, holidays and the general frivolity of the hazy, lazy days of summer. The time was one of reflection and angst at the vacuous void of this approach. I wondered, *Why this is happening to me? What would my life be like free of medicines? What is the reason for all this? What is the cause?* In these questions lies an inherent problem: today, we only look for the causality in healing. With causality, we end up a blind alley with only more causes being sought after.

> In the causal view of things, after all, every manifestation ultimately has a cause, and so it is not only permissible, but actually essential, to try to discover the cause of the cause ... but what it never leads to is any final conclusion. The ultimate cause of causes cannot be found.[2]

So, if the pursuit of cause is the road well trodden, how *should* we approach illness? Pursuing healing through the causality approach is, in fact, abdicating the responsibility to others, so that they may tell you what the problem is, and thus masking the real reason behind our state – using causality to hide from ourselves. Instead of looking at the cause, the more important area to be looking at is the information and intention of illness. This requires a deep introspective evaluation of yourself and everything about you. When suffering from an illness, it can seem like all the windows of light and opportunity are closing in and darkness has taken up residence in your life. It tests your character and every fibre of your being.

After my time in hospital undergoing treatment for cystic fibrosis, a lot changed in my thoughts towards health and how we

---

[2] Rudiger Dahlke and Thorwald Dethlefsen, *The Healing Power of Illness: The Meaning of Symptoms and How to Interpret Them*, Element Books Limited, 1997, p.66

are seduced by the quick-fix, instant panacea to remedy our bodies. We consume myriad health potions and pills to maintain vitality and never think any more about it. For so long, I was a passenger on this highway of health, hitch-hiking a ride from doctor to healer to physiotherapist to the next doctor. I was continuously hoping that someone would heal the physical manifestation of my illness, and that was when it dawned on me: only I could cure myself.

You can have all the treatments, take all the remedies and medication and visit all the top consultants in the world with no result. This leaves us feeling empty and castigated upon the rack of this cruel world. By looking at illness in this manner – as something outside our control that has singled us out, that we must battle and resist despite its menacing, magnetic mayhem – all we are doing is feeding it, and the illness refuses to leave. On the other hand, it is of utmost importance that you do not pigeonhole and box yourself in, or use illness as your ID card. I have never once classified myself as a person with cystic fibrosis, and I know that not doing that has helped me maintain my health at the level it is at. When you do not see illness as a foe, an important change takes place.

> When we learn to see our illness as companion or friend, it really does change the way the illness is present. The illness changes from a horrible intruder to a companion who has something to teach us. When we see what we have to learn form illness, then often the illness can gather itself and begin to depart.[3]

Edward Bach elaborates on this point further.

> Disease is in itself beneficent, and has for its object the bringing back of the personality to the divine will of the soul; and thus we can see that it is both preventable and avoidable, since if we could only realise for ourselves the mistakes we are making and correct these by spiritual and mental means there could be no need for the severe lessons of suffering.[4]

---

[3] John O'Donohue, *Eternal Echoes: Celtic Reflections on our Yearning to Belong*, Bantam Press, 2000, p.178
[4] Bach, *Heal Thyself*, p.9

These realisations were the building blocks that laid the foundations for my own healing.

When one flower blooms, it is spring everywhere.

A Zen monk

After a summer of seismic shifts, a ticket and trip to Brazil awaited me. A couple of months earlier, I had received a letter from Tony Clarkson, my godfather, regarding a healer called João de Deus. The letter spoke of amazing feats of healing that defied Western medical science. The seed of intent had been germinating since the letter had arrived, and this seed flowered and bloomed before me after my elongated stay in hospital. The letter, allied with the frustration of the summer just past, prompted me to act, and this saw Tony and I make our way to the small town of Abadiânia in central Brazil to seek this healer's help.

João de Deus (John of God)

A troubled youth tortured by a miraculous gift, João de Deus spent much of his life as a homeless person, travelling from one town to the next, helping the sick and ill in return for shelter and food. He would move onto the next town as soon as the local medic, dentist or priest took offence to his miraculous healing art and brought the heavy hand of the law crashing down on him. Fabrication and lies of the established hierarchies were charged against him and he was jailed on many occasions. Upon release, he would walk or beg a ride to a new city and so start his quest again. For many years he lived the vagabond lifestyle. After gruelling and punishing persecutions, he sought refuge in military barracks at Brasília as a civilian tailor (his father's profession). He traded many a year in the barracks, healing the sick and their families in return for protection. After nine years, the entities spoke to him, insisting that he could not limit himself to healing so few. With this guidance, he departed the safe environs of the barracks and used the money he'd saved to purchase a piece of land. The land purchased was extremely prosperous and contained emeralds, the worth of which allowed him to establish his centre in Abadiânia and begin a sanctuary of healing – the Casa de Dom Inácio.

Casa de Dom Inácio

The design of Casa de Dom Inácio (the House of St Ignatius Loyola) was inspired and named by João's principal entity: Dom Inácio.[5] It resembles a small hospital and is simply decorated. The simplicity of the decor masks the truly amazing healing energy of the place. The choice of site is due to many things: the natural energy of this part of Brazil, the solitude and also the fact that it is built on land rich in natural quartz, which in itself is a powerful energy source. The location is 'a source of fantastic energy which represents accumulations of pure energy where health and vitality is strengthened'.[6]

The house of Dom Inácio is open three days a week – Wednesday, Thursday and Friday – and opens at 7.30 a.m. on each of these days. The morning proceeds with a small introductory talk on the rules, regulations and protocol of the day. After the talk, a number of queues are formed (first-time queue, second-time queue, revision, and those with previously arranged operations) and the crowds disperse into their respective queue. Before the orientation talk, many shuffle to a number of blue-coated individuals outside, who help them translate their respective wishes into Portuguese to aid and facilitate a smooth flow of foot traffic before João de Deus.

The house is divided into a number of rooms that are all synergistically employed to aid and assist healing. The first of these rooms is the recovery room, where patients are taken after treatment for care and observation until they are strong enough to leave. This room contains twelve beds and the nurses are volunteers who provide compassionate care until the patient is

---

[5] An entity is a channelled consciousness of any kind, but generally a soul from the astral plane. Through João, spirit entities minister to the multitudes who come in search of a cure. João sits 'in-entity' (unconscious, taken over or 'overshadowed' by an entity from the spiritual plan), scans the patient, sees what they need and uses various healing methods to enable healing.

[6] Robert F Butts and Jane Roberts, *Seth Speaks: The Eternal Validity of the Soul*, Amber-Allen Publishing, USA, 1994

well enough to vacate. Adjacent to the recovery room is the first of two 'current' rooms. Inside these rooms, there are rows of people sitting on pews, lost in meditation and helping to raise the vibration and energy to assist João in doing his work. (In Edgar Cayce's *Atlantis*, there is reference to this type of combined energy as used by the Atlantians to achieve their extraordinarily advanced civilisation.) In the second room, there are more mediums and people meditating to raise the current in order to help João with his work. João also resides here in a chair as patients go before him for spiritual consultation. As soon as you enter the second current room, a powerful charge of energy courses through you for a split second as João scans your eyes and, with that, a snapshot synopsis of your lives (past and present) and well-being is taken. You are then directed whether you are to go for surgery, return to meditate or go for herbs. The final room of the Casa is the intensive operations room where those requiring long-term healing remain in a curative coma and where those who request invisible operations also go.

The Road to Abadiânia

> Improvement makes straight roads; but the crooked roads without improvement are roads of genius.
>
> William Blake

Four airports, a twenty-plus hour plane trip and a two-hour taxi ride and the destination of a small town high on the Goiás plateau of central Brazil, Abadiânia, is reached. Thousands flock daily to this beacon of hope and healing – the sick, the lame, the 'incurable' and the medically discarded – in search of a life free of suffering or illness. I joined this band of brothers and sisters and opened my heart, body and soul to the miracle of the Casa de Dom Inácio.

My first day before João de Deus was one of excitement, nervous churning and significance. My first visit was on 17 September 2003, my twenty-fifth birthday, a significant cornerstone and the start of a new chapter of health and enlightenment in my life. I remember the energy of nerves coursing through me, and the thoughts and hopes about the possible repercussions of the trip on my health. I'd read about the protocol, listened to many people speak about their experiences, viewed the websites and much more. However, it still did not prepare me for what I felt and bore witness to – a surreal healing environ surrounded by a congregation of people donned in white, early on the opening morning of the Casa and all united under the umbrella of compassion, love and light. The morning kicked off with an orientation followed by a powerful uniting of hands in saying the Lord's Prayer. The energy of the room beamed. Then we moved into our respective queues to go before João de Deus.

I remember passing through the first current room, full of people meditating and lost in a trance, facing their own inner battles and demons, while providing current and energy to João. Some faces were contorted with anguish and sadness; others were tinged with joy and serenity; while others lost their body to dance and swaying. A kind of cathartic cleansing was taking place for each and every one. The energy radiated throughout the first and second current room, feeding and energising the work that was to take place over the next couple of hours. The endless stream of people in their respective queues passed through the middle of the pews as each individual was spiritually prepared to meet João-in-entity.

Within seconds of entering the second current room where João-in-entity resided, a 'blueprint' of my physical and ethereal bodies was scanned. A sweeping sensation penetrated my body. It was like an instant snapshot, viewing my life (past and present), my current situation, my illness and my spiritual awareness.

As I approached João de Deus, the moment was incredibly fleeting – he wrote my prescription in a flowing foreign script and instructed me to go for surgery the next morning.

The next morning came quickly and with it the same protocol of moving into our respective queues. This time I entered the line for surgery. I was ushered past the two current rooms into a third room: the intensive operations room. This room has the dual purpose of caring for the long-term convalescents and also for those requesting invisible operations. Around the wall of this room was a line of beds where the long-term ill rested while an entity performed operations invisibly – paraplegics, leukaemia sufferers, AIDS sufferers and serious cancer patients were all being treated. Across the middle of the room, there were rows of benches, on which those requiring invisible operation sat, eyes closed, hands resting on their laps in meditation. Seated on the pews, I was given the instruction to close my eyes and uncross my legs and arms. For the entities to do their work, we were instructed to place our right hand over the area we wished to be operated and worked on. João entered the intensive operations room and, in one divine statement, he called for the operations to be completed. He declared the following: 'In the name of Jesus Christ, you are all operated. Let what needs to be done be done through me in the name of God.' At this time all operations necessary were completed internally, without visible surface scarring. Following these invisible operations, X-rays have shown that there are often small incisions and internal stitches.

Though not physically probed, sliced or diced, a sweeping, pre-med fatigue came over me. I remember holding the wall for support after the invisible surgery; my legs felt weak and my only thoughts were to get into my bed and stay there for the next twenty-four hours, as instructed. It is important to adhere to rest after invisible surgery, even more so than after conventional surgery. Due to the fact that many do not always feel the procedure completed, they think, to their folly, that they can continue free of rest. To disobey the importance of rest will result in the cessation of the healing process and, in some cases, worsen the condition.

My experience brought absolute fatigue and I was bedridden for the full twenty-four hours. The following morning I awoke afresh from my slumber with renewed hope and vigour, ready for the start of a new road to health. Several thoughts ran through my mind after this invisible surgery. Was this spiritual nirvana a 'window of opportunity' that had opened for me to start new beginnings? Then my mind began to consider what life might be like without cystic fibrosis. Would my character change? Would my approach to life change? Was I ready for this after years of

ias many miles to go. My visitations to Abadiânia
reak ranks with conventional medicine to a degree
it of my illness and embrace a more natural, non-
npowering practice, to the betterment of my
... in Abadiânia has opened me up to new healing
opportunities. I opened my heart and soul to change my health
and, with that, innumerable blessings came my way – meditation,
Buteyko breathing, magnetostimulation, energy medicine,
homeopathics, etc. Each of these have enlightened me and given
me more hope in the last few years than the previous twenty-five
years of allopathic medicine. Though this path to health has only
just begun, I feel that I now have the tools to conquer my ailment
and free me from a life of palliative medication.

Meditation

The power of surrendering, listening to your soul and taking
important time out to integrate with your soul, meditation
improves health by restoring and maintaining vital mental and
physical health. Bernie Siegel MD, a surgeon and professor at
Yale University, has written of the many marvellous benefits of
meditation.

> It tends to lower or normalise blood pressure, pulse rate and the
> levels of stress hormones in the blood. It produces changes in the
> brain wave patterns, showing less excitability ... meditation also
> raises pain threshold and reduces one's biological age ... in short,
> it reduces wear and tear on both body and mind, helping people
> live a better and longer.[7]

I practise a very simple yet empowering meditation exercise every
day for as little as 15–20 minutes.

It is an inner-body meditation – a meditation that allows me to
communicate with my body and influence my cellular make-up
through surrounding my body and cells with a healing, positive
environment. After reading Dr Bruce Lipton's *The Biology of Belief*
and understanding the field of epigenetics (the idea that our cells

---

[7] B S Siegel, *Love, Medicine and Miracles*, Arrow Books, 1988

are strongly influenced by our environment), I believe we hold a tool – a simple, empowering tool – to better our health: using our environment, not our genetics to shape our health.

Simply begin breathing. Relax your body with each and every breath and breathe out energies that do not serve your body. As you are doing this, also breathe in healing energies from a source – visualise a healing light and see that light cocoon your body, growing and glowing with each breath.

Then, begin to direct your breath to each part of your body, starting with your feet. Feel your feet and feel a warm glow around your feet. Then move up toward your ankles, lower limbs, knees, upper limbs and on and on till you reach the crown of your head. Along each point of your body, direct healing energies towards that body part. Sit holding attention to each body part for as long as feels comfortable.

Practice makes perfect. Healing will come when we consistently dedicate ourselves to nurturing our life energy. Release and let go of frustrating experiences and know that it is just perfect. Diligence and dedication can overcome all.

BUTEYKO BREATHING

The Art of Breathing Less and Living Longer[8]

Shut your mouth and save your life.

George Catlin

Breath of Life

Our first breath is our most important. However, many births today are clocked to the timetable of the hospital, not nature. From the safety and comfort of the womb, the child is delivered into chaos – bright lights, surgical masks, loud noises, etc. The umbilical cord is severed within moments of delivery, forcing the child into a fight-and-flight strategy. The umbilical cord is of great importance to the child, as it supplies the required oxygen to the brain. As Michael Sky has said, 'The transition from breathing with the umbilical cord to breathing with the lungs must be as smooth and uninterrupted as possible.'[9]

Oxygen deprivation can lead to serious repercussions for the child's health. The uncut cord can continue to provide oxygen throughout the labour and should support each other until the child ceases to employ it, allowing the child to effectively cut his own cord. The birthing process is the child's first introduction into this world and the process could not be more frightening.

Breathing is an unconscious process, something we take for granted, an automatic course that begins at birth and continues till our last breath on earth. This unconscious action never crosses any healthy person's mind. However, for those who are respira-

---

[8] My thanks go to Charles Maguire for his efforts in editing and compiling material for some sections of this chapter.

[9] Michael Sky, *Breathing: Expanding Your Power and Energy*, Bear & Company, UK, 1990, p.57

torally challenged, our breath is paramount to our well-being. The breathing method we adopt is vital to our quality of life.

Buteyko Breathing

And the Lord God formed man of the dust of the ground, and breathed into his nostrils the breath of life; and man became a living soul.

Genesis 2:7, King James Bible

The art of breathing less and living longer resonated with me quickly. After twenty-five years of conventional physiotherapy treatment and never any real relief attained, the invitation to attend a Buteyko breathing workshop was a refreshing, self-empowering few days that revolutionised my approach to breath inhalation and exhalation.

I can remember clearly the morning prior to the workshop. I was being put through my paces with my daily aerobics – a morning session would usually entail an hour of respiration exercises. This all included the usual cacophony of constant coughing, nausea-inducing asphyxiation and trips to the bathroom, where I'd hug the toilet bowl as if I'd been out on a serious drinking bender the night before. The harshness of my coughing caused a constant feeling of nausea and turned me a nice shade of beetroot.

The application of this physical therapy was a continuous self-defeating cycle as the process of perpetual clearance is a losing battle – the more I coughed, the more congested I got. The creation of excess mucus is simply the body's defence against loss of carbon dioxide. By reducing our breathing, the body auto-regulates itself and the spasms of coughing subside considerably.

Conventional treatment for cystic fibrosis includes a whole range of breathing tests. The lung-function tests (also called pulmonary function tests or PFTs) evaluate how well your lungs work. The tests determine how much air your lungs can hold, how quickly you can move air in and out of your lungs and how well your lungs put oxygen into and remove carbon dioxide from your blood. These tests can diagnose lung disease, measure the severity of lung problems and check to see how well treatment for a lung disease is working.

Spirometry is the first lung-function test done. It measures how much and how quickly you can move air out of your lungs. For this test, you breathe into a mouthpiece attached to a recording device (spirometer). The information collected by the spirometer may be printed out on a chart called a spirogram. The more common lung-function values measured with spirometry are:

- FORCED VITAL CAPACITY (FVC): This measures the amount of air you can exhale with force after you inhale as deeply as possible.

- FORCED EXPIRATORY VOLUME (FEV): This measures the amount of air you can exhale with force in one breath. The amount of air you exhale may be measured at one second (FEV1), two seconds (FEV2) or three seconds (FEV3). FEV1 divided by FVC can also be determined.

- FORCED EXPIRATORY FLOW 25–75%: This measures the air flow halfway through an exhale (FVC).

- PEAK EXPIRATORY FLOW (PEF): This measures how quickly you can exhale. It is usually measured at the same time as your forced vital capacity (FVC).

- MAXIMUM VOLUNTARY VENTILATION (MVV): This measures the greatest amount of air you can breathe in and out during one minute.

The use of these tests and, in particular, of FE1s involved great inhalations of breath and exhaling with every sinew of strength my lungs could muster. I felt I was running on empty. On completion I would be left a puce-like colour and fatigued, which very often led to more coughing! Such tests are a rather crude form of gauging the wellness of someone's lung health, especially as the method involves the antithesis of Buteyko breathing – *deep breathing*. I will discuss this in more detail later in this chapter.

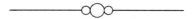

CURRY SPICE COULD ALLEVIATE CYSTIC FIBROSIS

Researchers from Yale University have tested a curry spice – turmeric – on mice and have been finding that administering low doses of a component of the spice can make most of the symptoms of cystic fibrosis disappear. Michael Caplan, part of the Yale research team, is quoted in *New Scientist* saying, 'It can almost completely correct the measurable defects of the disease.'

Cystic fibrosis is passed on when two copies of the defective gene CTFR are inherited. The outcome is that an important protein is misfolded, trapping the protein from the cell surface, therefore making it difficult for salt to move in and out of the cells. The end result is that mucus in both the airways and the digestive tract becomes thick and sticky, trapping bacteria that is incapable of being released through the nose and mouth and nutrients are unable to be absorbed.

Caplan and his research team reasoned that if you could somehow unfold the misshapen protein and allow it to get to the cell surface, you may be able to greatly assist the condition of cystic fibrosis sufferers.

Research undertaken at the University of Toronto has shown that, 'curcumin, a component of turmeric, makes it possible for protein to escape to the cell surface by starving the inspector proteins of calcium'. With this information, the Yale research team decided to test turmeric on mice with a disorder similar to cystic fibrosis. The outcome and results were promising with improvements to the animals' gut problems and, 'changes in the electrical potential across the nasal epithelium', which suggested improvements in the respiratory system.

With the knowledge provided from the Yale research team, the US Cystic Fibrosis Foundation is starting a human clinical trial. Neil Sweezey, from the Hospital for Sick Children in Toronto has said, 'One reason for optimism is that you may not need to get much of the protein working to significantly improve a patient's health.'[10]

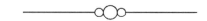

The History of Buteyko

Konstantin Pavlovich Buteyko is the founding father of Buteyko breathing. A passion for understanding the complexities of the human organism and how it worked propelled Konstantin Buteyko into the field of medicine. As a medical student, he was assigned to observe the breathing patterns of ill patients. After hundreds of hours of observation, he noticed a considerable and uniformed deepening of breath when death neared. Through recording these notable differences in breath, he was able to predict with accuracy the days or hours that each patient under his supervision had left before death. The outcome of these results shaped Buteyko's future.

He observed that breathing patterns were closely allied with the extent of the illness and began to ponder this further. He found that overbreathing lowered carbon-dioxide levels in the body. He hypothesised that if low levels of carbon dioxide were caused by overbreathing then, by correcting breathing patterns, he could possibly cure the presenting respiratory ailment.

The above hypothesis was put to the test and the outcome after testing his theory on sufferers of asthma, stenocardia and other diseases proved the theory. In each and every patient,

---

[10] See: Alison Motluk, 'Curry spice could alleviate cystic fibrosis', *New Scientist.com* news service, 22 April 2004

symptoms disappeared and normalised once their breathing pattern was corrected, normalising their carbon-dioxide shortfall. When asked to return to initial breathing style, symptoms returned quickly. The outcome of this proved that hyperventilation causes a depletion of carbon dioxide; low levels of carbon dioxide in the organism cause blood vessels to spasm and also cause oxygen starvation of the tissues. This results in a whole range of 'defence mechanisms' that have been previously misunderstood and labelled as diseases.

Deep Breathing

The breath of life was breathed into man's nostrils.

Individuals very poorly understand the importance of, and correct approach to, breathing. Breathing is life itself. It is strongly connected to health. Today, there is a plethora of disease – it is rife among our civilisation. It is commonplace. Why is this? The answer is inhalation through the mouth. Humans are the only mammal that *mouth-breathes* – one of the primary causes of disease.

The mouth of man, as well as that of the brutes, was made for the reception and mastication of food for the stomach, and other purposes; but the nostrils with their delicate and fibrous linings for purifying and warming the air in its passage, have been mysteriously constructed, and designed to stand guard over the lungs – to measure the air and equalise its draughts, during hours of repose.

The atmosphere is nowhere near pure enough for man's breathing until it has passed through this mysterious refining process; and therefore the imprudence and danger of admitting it an unnatural way, in double quantities, upon the lungs, and charged with the surrounding epidemic or contagious infections of the moment.[11]

---

[11] George Catlin, *Shut Your Mouth and Save Your Life*, London, N Truebner and Co., 1870, p.10

The nostrils have fine little hairs on the inside of your nose – cilia – which filter and warm the incoming air before it moves through to the lungs. The lungs require a warm, moist environment and it is therefore essential that the air drawn in meets this requirement. Viktor Schauberger goes further to say that 'it is vital that the characteristic inner temperature of each of the millions of micro-organisms contained in the macro-organisms be maintained'.[12]

In France, for example, investigations have shown that the air in the streets of Paris, which is warmer than normal air, contains 36,000 pathogenic bacteria per cubic metre, whereas in the forest and over the fields this reduced very sharply to only 490 airborne germs per cubic metre – 0.0136% of the above figure.[13] Other data also infers a correlation between green space and disease, as exemplified by comparative levels of tuberculosis in relation to the population of three major European cities set out below:[14]

London	14% green space	1.9% tuberculosis
Berlin	10% green space	2.2% tuberculosis
Paris	4.5% green space	4.1% tuberculosis

These facts alone show the detriment of mouth-breathing to our health through the harmful bacteria that is ingested, and also clearly shows the importance of cilia in preventing over-saturation of the air getting to the lungs and forming our defence against foreign particles. The Buteyko method adheres to this principle.

Years of conventional schooling in physiotherapy, FE1s, peak flows and other such tests caused me much frustration, born out of a perpetual losing battle with my lungs in my twenties. The inhalation and exhalation of physio would leave me gasping. Physio was serving me no purpose.

Prior to finding out about the Buteyko method of breathing, I went through several breathing exercises to aid and alleviate my

---

[12] Viktor Schauberger, 'The Forest and its Significance (Der Wald und seine Bedeutung)', *Tau Magazine*, vol. 146, p.2; Callum Coats, *Living Energies: An Exposition of Concepts Related to the Theories of Viktor Schauberger*, Gateway, Second Edition, USA, 2002, p.105

[13] Coats, *Living Energies*, p.106

[14] Gro Harlem Brundtland, *Our Common Future*, Oxford University Press, 1998

breathing. One episode I remember was after my lung had collapsed. The doctor gave me blowing apparatus and asked me to take a deep breath in through the mouthpiece. As I exhaled, I was to move air-like balls into the air and hold them there for as long as possible. The aim was to hold the three balls in the air all at once, to govern the well-being of my lungs. Other exercises involved taking very big breaths in through the nose and out through the mouth into the FE1 machine, while placing a nasal clip on my nose during exhalation. Just these two methods alone are converse to Buteyko's principles and most likely exacerbate rather than help the person with the respiratory problem. This crude form of respiratory exercise worsened my state and brought about spasms of coughing and a feeling of disappointment that this gauge for lung capacity was further damaging the health of my lungs.

> Forceful exhaling causes too much carbon dioxide to be carried out with each breath. A forced breath out results in the subsequent inhalation being large. This loss of carbon dioxide will cause spasm of smooth muscle, increased mucus and can lead to an asthma attack. An estimated 80 percent of asthma sufferers will experience an attack from big breathing within two minutes. It is logical therefore to conclude that breathing exercises involving big breathing will produce the same symptoms in a relatively short period of time. Instead of increasing lung capacity, these exercises will lead to increased mucus and spasms causing airway obstruction.
>
> Another misguided practice involves forceful removal of mucus with coughing exercises or tapping of the back. Mucus is part of the body's defence mechanism against the loss of carbon dioxide. Forcibly removing mucus results in increased breathing causing a loss of carbon dioxide. This will create more mucus. To remove mucus practice reduced breathing exercises and sniff up a mixture of warm water with a half teaspoon of sea salt dissolved in it. (An alternative is to drink a glass of warm water with a quarter teaspoon of sea salt dissolved in it, but some people find this too severe).[15]

---

[15] Patrick G McKeown, *Asthma Free Naturally: Everything You Need to Know About Taking Control of your Asthma*, Harper Thorsons, London, 2005, p.76

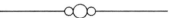

HIMALAYAN CRYSTAL SALT – THE ESSENCE OF LIFE

With reference to Patrick McKeown's book, *Asthma Free Naturally*, and the theory of consuming sea salt to reduce mucus, the best form of sea salt I've had the good fortune to use is Himalayan crystal sea salt.

For millions of years, through the unrelenting out-pouring of energy from the sun, our oceans have slowly been evaporated as part of the water cycle. The residue of this evaporation has left behind a vast pool of solar energy within the sea salt. For over 250 million years the salt has remained untapped... until now. The salt comes from a time when our planet was a pristine ecosystem. Containing eighty-four minerals and trace elements essential to our health and well-being, the salt is truly an elixir of life.

This is unlike its industrially processed cousin, sodium chloride, where the unnatural man-made crystals are isolated from each other with no life-giving energy properties. In fact, the body must use up huge amounts of its own reserves of energy to break them down. With the Himalayan sea salt, the crystals are harmoniously connected to each other, meaning the salt is perfectly balanced and easily metabolised by the body. The crystal is the antithesis of sodium chloride and full of life energy. The net result of this salt is the positive effects in changing the state of respiratory system, circulatory, organ and connective tissue and nervous system functions.

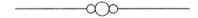

CAYENNE PEPPER

I have employed the use of cayenne, as it is a natural expectorant as well as an anti-inflammatory for the lungs. I dilute a little cayenne in water and drink it.

Cayenne can be used in a host of different areas with equally beneficial results. Cayenne is rich in vitamin C. It is considered thermogenic, meaning it can speed up metabolism and assist in weight loss. It also improves circulation. Try putting a bit of cayenne between your shoes and socks on a cold winter's day – it helps to keep the feet warm. Cayenne also helps to relieve pain, not only due to its endorphin-enhancing properties but also because, when it is diluted and used topically, it helps to block the transmission of Substance P, which transports pain messages to the brain.

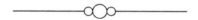

The Theory behind Buteyko

The premise behind Buteyko is the importance of the biological role of carbon dioxide in the human organism. To sustain the normal biochemical processes of the human organism, a definite concentration of 7% carbon dioxide is needed.

The problem facing the human organism has been as a result of the loss of carbon dioxide in our atmosphere. The human body has countered this loss by creating its own internal air environment within the alveolar of the lungs. The internal air environment is 6.5% carbon dioxide. Interestingly, 7–8% of the gaseous mix in the womb is also made up of 7–8% carbon dioxide.

Professor Buteyko delivered his findings on this subject to the World Congress of Biochemistry in Moscow in 1972 stating the following:

1. Carbon dioxide is, through the conversion into carbonic acid, the most important buffer system in the body's regulation of its acid–base balance (acid–alkali balance). A low level of carbon dioxide may lead to alkalosis. If the level of carbon dioxide lowers below 3%, shifting the pH to 8, then the whole organism dies.

2. A low level of carbon dioxide causes a displacement of the oxyhemoglobin dissociation curve, thereby not allowing correct oxygenation of the tissues and vital organs (Bohr effect).

3. Poor oxygenation leads to hypoxia and a whole gamut of medical disorders.

4. Carbon dioxide is a smooth muscle vessel dilator. Therefore a shortfall of carbon dioxide causes spasming of the brain tissue and bronchus tissue, etc.

5. Hyperventilation causes a progressive loss of carbon dioxide. The higher the breathing rate, the lower the carbon dioxide level.

6. Carbon dioxide is the catalyst for the body's metabolic processes, playing a vital role in biosynthesis of amino acids and their amides, lipids, carbohydrates, etc.

The physiological effects of breathing less are clearly stated by Professor Buteyko. His maxim of 'breathe less' is vital for good health. Overbreathing places undue pressure on the human body and leads to a carbon dioxide deficit. In 1909, an experiment was carried out by a leading and well-respected physiologist of the time, Dr Henderson, which showed the detriments of deep breathing. In his experiments, animals were mechanically induced to breathe deeply and death was the result.[16]

---

[16] For a more comprehensive analysis of the physiological role of carbon dioxide, see VA Kazarinov, 'The Biochemical Basis of K P Buteyko's Theory of Disease of Deep Respiration', in *Buteyko Method: Experience of Implementation in Medical Practice*, ed. by K P Buteyko, Moscow, Patriot Press, 1990

The Importance of Carbon Dioxide to the Body

- THE BOHR EFFECT: learning to reduce breathing. Reduced breathing allows more carbon dioxide to stay in the system. This leads to better oxygenation of all the body's cells and tissues which in turn leads to all the organs to function more effectively and efficiently.

- ACID–ALKALI BALANCE: through the conversion into carbonic acid, carbon dioxide is the most vital player in maintaining the body's acid–base balance. Lowering of carbon dioxide in the body can result in a more alkaline system, making the body more susceptible to virus and allergies.

- THE NERVOUS SYSTEM: lowering of carbon dioxide in the nerve cells heightens the threshold of their excitability, awakening all sensitive stimulus of the nervous system and resulting in irritability, increased anxiety attacks, insomnia, allergies, etc. In conjunction with this, the breathing centre in the brain is stimulated, creating further depletion of carbon dioxide in the body. A perpetual self-defeating, self-induced circle is started.

The Control Pause

The exercise that I have used to great effect has been the control pause. This requires inhalation of breath for two seconds, followed by exhalation of breath for roughly three seconds, both from your nose. You then clamp your nasal cavities and hold for as long as is comfortable. The longer and more comfortably you can hold your breath demonstrates the level of carbon dioxide in the alveoli. It is important to bear in mind that this is a measure of carbon dioxide levels in the body, and not a way to increase carbon dioxide levels.

TO PERFORM THE CONTROL PAUSE

- Take just over twenty minutes for yourself in a quiet space. Sit relaxed and upright.

- Inhale for two seconds and exhale for three seconds. Using a stopwatch, record the time that you can comfortably hold your breath for. Do not pressure your respiratory system to hold longer than is comfortable, as that will set back the results you are trying to achieve – a gasp of breath after holding for so long will result in loss of carbon dioxide.

- Follow the Buteyko principle of 'breathing less' for five or so minutes.

- Proceed again and measure the control pause. On each occasion, your CP should incrementally improve. Follow again with reduced breathing for five minutes and repeat this process for two more reduced breathing intervals of five minutes.

At the beginning, my control pause was quite low – equating to a low, fixed level of carbon dioxide in my body. Consequently, I was inhaling a large volume of air in order to maintain this level. Though it has taken time to re-educate my breathing patterns, breaking the habit of overbreathing was most important for my well-being. I regularly employ this exercise, at least twice a day and three or even four times a day when I am feeling unwell. It is a simple, non-invasive exercise that brings good health to my lungs.

The exercise has helped me relinquish my two inhalers – serotide and ventolin – and has helped me reduce from five nebulisers a day to two – all in the space of a few years. Bountiful benefits have blessed me since I have employed Buteyko breathing and the control pause exercise. My energy levels have soared stratospherically. One day I managed to play twenty-five holes of golf and not lose breath or produce a single bead of perspiration. I then played competitive tennis later that evening! I finished stronger and felt better than my supposedly healthy opponent! My quality of sleep has improved, as has my general well-being. I am no longer as nauseous when doing my exercises and I have fewer headaches from the harshness of my coughing. I even have improved time management – no longer losing an hour in the morning and evening to perpetual clearance exercises. Two twenty-minute control pause exercise sets give me a whole lot more time to myself.

Another note that I must share about the control pause is that it has also become the test for what is good for my body and what is not. My breathing would become quite erratic on the ingestion of too much protein – for example, after the consumption of my 'Micky steak sandwich special': steak, peppers, onions and cheese, all smothered in mustard and ketchup and served in a heated baguette – a veritable feast. That will be sorely missed from my menu. Foods such as this would considerably alter my breathing pattern and would, at times, trigger a bout of coughing. My breathing pattern and my use of the control pause is a perfect and accurate indicator for what is good or a hindrance for my body.

Though I am still developing this technique, the benefits of the last couple of years and thoughts of the future benefits of Buteyko has given me hope and belief that this debilitating, genetic disease affecting over 900 families in Ireland can be assuaged and alleviated through this self-empowering breathing exercise.

Buteyko Technique

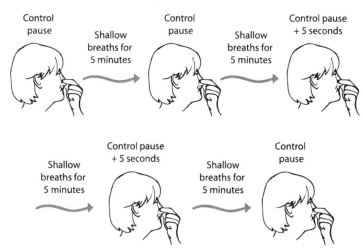

Practise this three times a day before meals until your symptoms disappear

Ailments and Disease Caused by Overbreathing

acidosis/alkalosis

agoraphobia*

allergies*

anaemia*

angina*

anorexia nervosa*

anxiety

apathy

arthritis*

asthma

bedwetting

breathlessness

bronchitis

bulimia*

cancer*

cerebral palsy*

chest pains*

chronic rhinitis

chronic diarrhoea

chronic fatigue syndrome*

chronic pneumonia*

circulation problems*

colds

concentration problems

constipation

coughing

cystic fibrosis*

depression*

deterioration of hearing

deterioration of sight

diarrhoea

drug addiction*

dry skin

eczema

emphysema*

epilepsy*

fear

flu

flatulence

hay fever

headaches

heart attacks*

heart conditions*

heartburn

hyperventilation

impotence

infertility*

insomnia*

irritability

IBS

irregular heartbeat

itching

kidney disease*

memory loss

MS*

muscular pains

muscular spasms

nightmares*

oedema*

painful and irregular periods*

palpitations*

panic attacks

Parkinson's disease

PMS*

short temper

shortness of breath

skin problems*

sleep apnoea*

snoring

sterility*

stomach sickness

stress

stroke*

thyroid problems

tinnitus*

Type 1 diabetes*

Ulcers*

varicose veins*

weight loss*

weight gain*

★

This list represents only some of the ailments and diseases that Professor Buteyko found to be caused by overbreathing. More than 90% of the population suffers from one or more of the conditions shown on the list. When Professor Buteyko treated his clients for overbreathing, their conditions either improved or disappeared completely. However, for the asterisked ailments, it is strongly advised that you consult your doctor before attending a qualified Buteyko practitioner.

WEEKLY RECORD KEEPING CHART

Time	Control Pause	Shallow Breath	Control Pause	Shallow Breath	Control Pause +5 seconds	Shallow Breath	Control Pause +5 seconds	Shallow Breath	Control Pause	Medication Intake & Physical Condition
MORNING										
AFTERNOON										
EVENING										
MORNING										
AFTERNOON										
EVENING										
MORNING										
AFTERNOON										
EVENING										
MORNING										
AFTERNOON										
EVENING										
MORNING										
AFTERNOON										
EVENING										
MORNING										
AFTERNOON										
EVENING										
MORNING										
AFTERNOON										
EVENING										

Dear Mike,

Many congratulations on the ball, it was brilliant. Our friends said it was the best they can remember.

I was talking to Ed last night about an extraordinary experience a colleague of mine had last week.

His name is Dr J E and his doctorate is in psychology. He is a trainer of psychotherapy and has written several books.

He went to Brazil with a medical doctor to see a Brazilian healer. The pair of them were going to see this healer for their own private reasons.

What they saw astounded them and defied every belief that they had around medicine and healing. The GP doctor broke down as what he saw went in the face of a lifetime of training and practising medicine.

The psychic healer sees three or four hundred people per day and the location of the healing centre is so positioned because of a natural bedrock of crystal under the site. This keeps the energies high.

The healer evidently leaves his body and spirit guides come into his body. J said that as the next person in the queue moved to see him, the eyes of the healer could change colour as a new spirit guide came in.

This letter was the map that began my path less conventional.

When it is your turn, you have to have clear in your mind what it is your want, and that's all. He said that the voice, through the healer, knows everything about you.

From that face to face, and then the subsequent passing you on to other psychic people, operations were performed invisibly and people who were blind could then see, people with tumours were having tumours removed, people in wheelchairs were getting up and walking.

Please appreciated this is second hand from a friend (and an extremely logical person), but I thought that I would like to share this with you, and it might be that it is of interest to you, or even to speak to my colleague direct.

If you would like to follow it up, please contact me and I will help you.

Lots of love,
Tony and Sheila

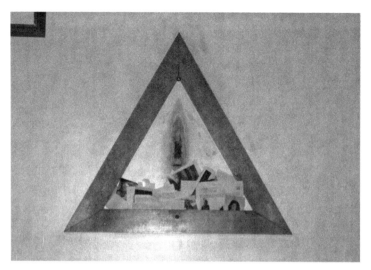

The Triangle – a powerful symbol of the Casa. The Brazilian World Cup Squad was blessed by João de Deus before heading to World Cup 2002. Note Ronaldo's hairdo – the shaved triangle on his forehead

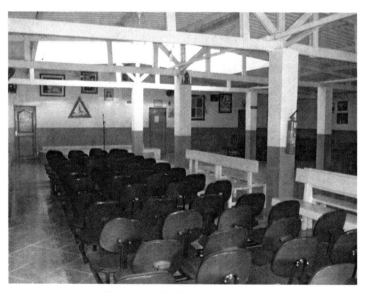

The main hall of Casa Dom Inácio

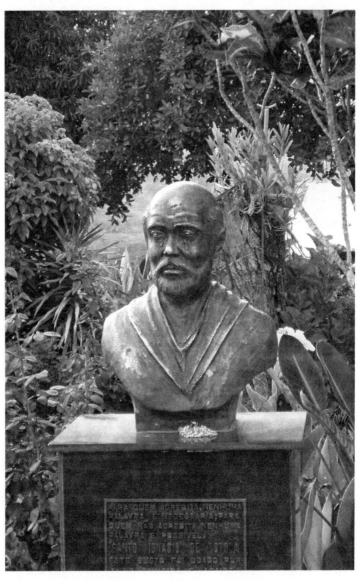

The bronze bust of Dom St Ignatius

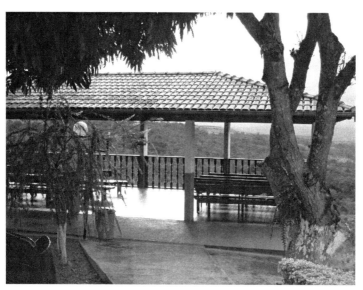

The veranda overlooking the leafy green valley of Abadânia

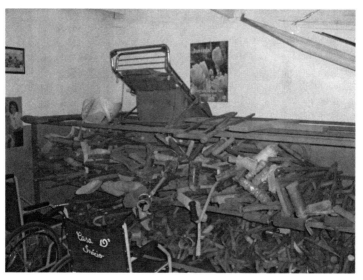

*Discarded wheelchairs, sticks and so on after their visits before João.
Many leave them behind after seeing the Miracle Man*

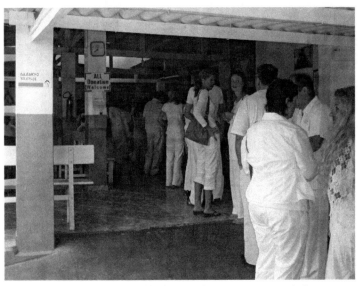

Dressed in white, a band of brothers and sisters queue to go before João de Deus

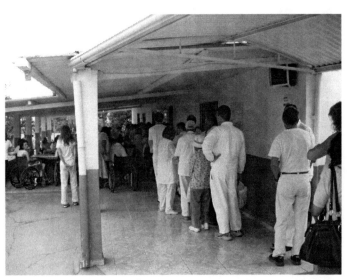

Soup is served every day for all who attend the Casa. It is part of the healing ritual. This is the daily queue that forms outside the Casa for the soup

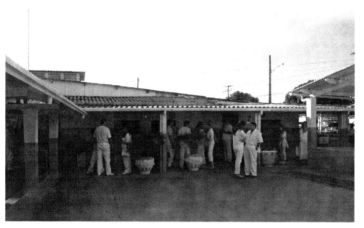

Meeting with the translators before going in front of João de Deus

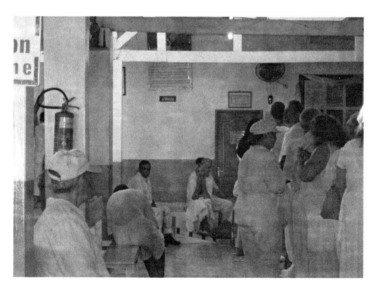

Waiting in the main room to take their seats in current to help raise the vibrations and engergies for João de Deus' work

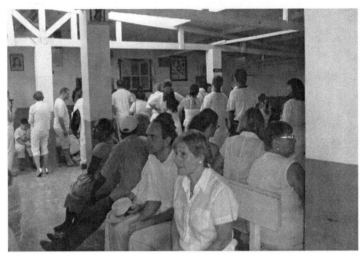

Waiting for João de Deus in the main hall

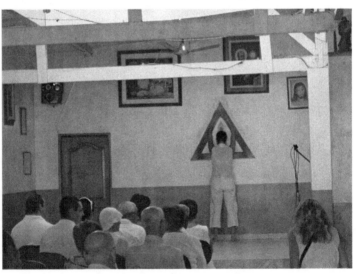

Many people pray before the triangle

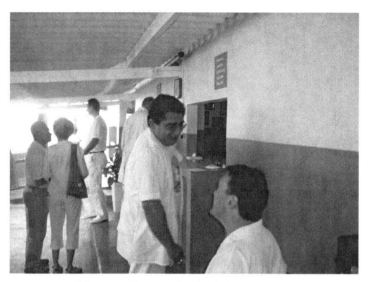

One of the many blue-coated individuals assisting the Casa

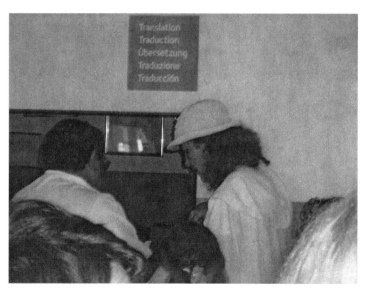

Translation lines. These lines help people get their requests translated into Portugese before going before João de Deus

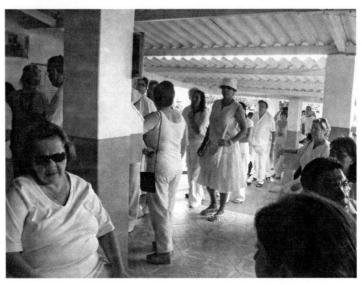

People shuffle into their respective lines before going before João de Deus

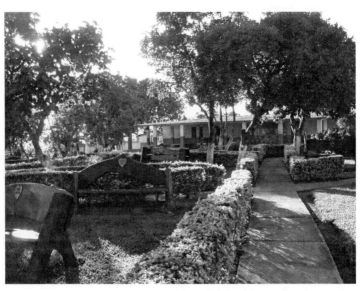

The gardens of Casa Dom Inácio

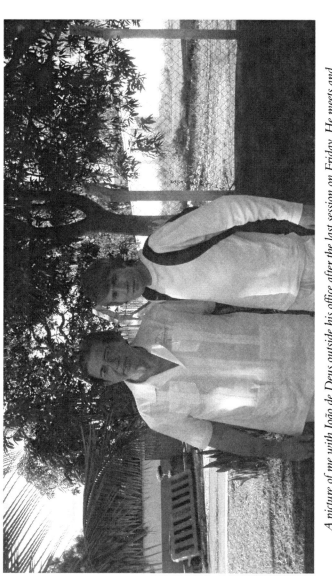

A picture of me with João de Deus outside his office after the last session on Friday. He meets and poses for photos with groups and individuals after every Friday session

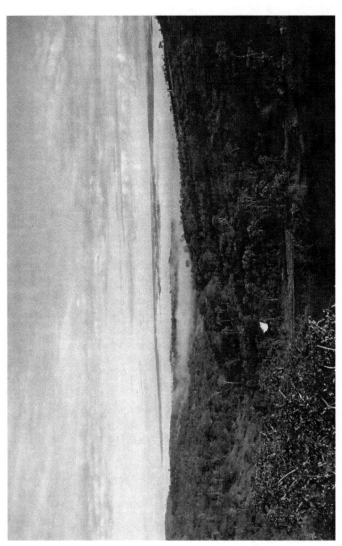

The green valleys of Abadânia and the smoky haze of lowland fog

ENERGY
Medicine of the Future

Our remedies oft in ourselves do lie.

William Shakespeare
All's Well That Ends Well

Energy medicine is defined as the use of the body's own innate healing properties to return us to physical and emotional homeostasis. We are returning to and honouring the ancient ways of healing with the employment of energy medicine. For over 5,000 years, the Chinese have understood and used the healing energies of the body. The Chinese discovered a complex system of energy lines that run throughout the body and these meridian points form the foundation for their healing practices.

In energy medicine, 'energy is both the medicine, and energy is also the patient'.[1] The body's healing is naturally activated, helping you restore lost energies that have been weakened, disturbed or put out of balance. You become your own physician and as such you are in control of your own healing. As mentioned in chapter one, too often we hand over responsibility to others for our healing, and with that we give away our *own* power for healing. Energy medicine allows us to cultivate the sensitive energies from within, and helps us to realise the powerful panacea that exists inside all of us.

The body is 'designed by the creator to live for twenty and one-half periods of seven years, or about 144 years. Our failure to do this is the result of our inability to live within the laws of

---

[1] Donna Eden and David Feinstein, *The Energy Medicine Kit*, Sounds True, Kit Edition, USA, 2005, p.9

39

f the body to overcome illness and maintain
e's most amazing and remarkable feats.
day run counter to the laws of nature.
proper nutrition, a sedentary lifestyle
ne body out of a natural environ of health.
eas in energy medicine will provide the body
d food to heal itself.

tonian vs Einsteinian Medicine

Today our school of medicine is dictated by Newton and his model of viewing the make-up of the human body as a 'divine mechanism' that can be stripped down, oiled and replaced via surgery or pharmacologic means. This approach to medicine views every piece of the body as mechanical process. The heart, for instance, is seen as a motorised pump that delivers oxygen and blood to the organ systems of the body and the brain. Western medicine thinks that it can better the process and creations of nature, and replace an ailing heart with a mechanical copy of the heart by mimicking the functional qualities. The advances of biomedical technology may allow more spare parts to be used, but sadly draws medicine away from the understanding of an illness. Instead of confronting the illness and understanding the information it is presenting, we ingest countless drugs or reroute the problem via surgery. Western and Newtonian medicine believes that the sum of the parts make up the whole, and with this there is a guiding light belief that you can manipulate the parts of the body to bring health to the whole. However, this principle or belief is very limiting, as it ignores the incredible latticework of interwoven energies that make up the vital forces of the body. Here's where medicine needs to re-evaluate its field and look to Einstein and his formula – $E = MC^2$ – for the medicine of the twenty-first century.

Matter is energy and follows energy – this formula forms the foundation that we are all beings of energy. Through the creation of good, flowing energy we can create good health for ourselves.

---

[2] S D McCune and N J Milanovich, *The Light Shall Set You Free*, Athena Publishing, 1996

Instead of conventional means of treatment, energy medicine employs the body's own energy to bring vital forces back. With energy medicine:

> the energetic network, which represents the physical/cellular framework, is organised and nourished by 'subtle' energetic systems which coordinate the life force with the body. There is a hierarchy of subtle energetic systems that coordinate electro-physiologic and hormonal function as well as cellular structure within the physical body. It is primarily from these subtle levels that health and illness originate.[3]

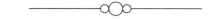

ENERGY EXERCISE – THE THREE THUMPS

Harmony can be restored to the body through a variety of 'energises'. Donna Eden discusses the idea that tapping certain points on the body can 'activate a sequence of responses that will restore you when you are tired, increase your vitality, and keep your immune system strong amid stress'.[4] She refers to these points as 'The Three Thumps'.

1. K–27: the K–27 is the twenty-seventh point of the kidney meridian. Exercising this point via tapping will stimulate good energy around the body, release negative thought patterns and bring you focus when you have difficulty concentrating. Place your right hand on your collarbone and run your thumb and middle finger towards each other until they meet at the U-point of the collarbone. Then, run both

---

[3] Richard Gerber MD, *Vibrational Medicine: The #1 Handbook of Subtle-Energy Therapies*, Bear & Company, UK, 2001, p.43

[4] Donna Eden and David Feinstein, *Energy Medicine: Balance your Body's Energies for Optimum Health, Joy and Vitality*, Penguin, SA, 2000, p.63

your thumb and middle finger down an inch from the U-point and out an inch. Both finger and thumb should fall into a natural groove in your chest cavity – the location of the K-27 point. On finding this location, tap the point with your finger and thumb for a period of twenty seconds. This point is great to use if you are tired at work – an excellent way to combat the 'three o'clock slump'!

2. THYMUS: tapping the thymus gland will boost your immune system, increase strength and vitality, and stimulate all your energies. The thymus is located an inch or two below the K-27 towards the centre of the sternum. I use this point and the spleen points religiously when I feel the effects of a cold coming on. Again, tap the point for a period of twenty seconds.

3. SPLEEN POINTS: tapping your spleen points is a quick way to boost your energy levels, balance blood chemistry in the body and strengthen the immune system. The spleen is:

   ...central to the functioning of the immune system. Tapping your spleen's neurolymphatic reflex points serves to synchronise your body's rhythms, harmonise its energies and its hormones, remove toxins, fight infection, combat general malaise during or after stress, counter dizziness, modulate blood chemistry and better metabolise food.[5]

Moving down an inch from the thymus point and out two to three inches (below your nipples), you will find the location of the spleen points. Tap here for a period of twenty seconds.

---

[5] Eden and Feinstein, *Energy Medicine*, pp.67–8

I use these points on a daily basis to create good energy in my body. They help me reduce the severity and frequency of colds and infections through gentle self-empowering non-invasive means. These exercises consume a little over a minute of your time and can be administered as frequently as you like without side effects or harm to your body.

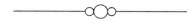

Homoeopathy

The medicine of the future needs to be more than the sum of each part. The future needs to embrace a more holistic, 360 ° view.

> The trend toward 'holism' in medicine will ultimately move physicians toward the recognition that, in order for human beings to experience health, they must enjoy an integrated relationship between body, mind and soul.[6]

One such field, homoeopathy, takes this holistic viewpoint and takes account of more than just the physical symptoms in the search for an appropriate cause. Samuel Hahnemann is the founding father of homoeopathy. Hahnemann was a brilliant physician who became disillusioned and dissatisfied with the journey that medicine was taking. He based his treatment on the principle that 'like cures like'. The 'Law of Similars' was the premise that what produced symptoms of ill health in a healthy individual could provide cure in a sick person. The most famous example was the employment of cinchona (china bark) in the treatment of malaria. Taking into account the principle of 'like cures like', cinchona was ideal for treating malaria as it reproduced the symptoms of malaria in someone who was healthy. Its success lay in its ability to reproduce the patients' 'total symptom complex' in an otherwise healthy individual. This process

---

[6] Gerber, *Vibrational Medicine*, p.66

activated the body's own defence system to bring about healing.

My first encounter with energy medicine was homoeopathy. My father is a classical homoeopath and the access to that knowledge changed our family's view of medicine. In 1997, I entered University College Dublin. I was preparing for exams in the library, gently rocking my chair back and forth while studying my materials for an upcoming Christmas exam, when I suddenly rocked my chair too far back and lost my balance. In doing so, I fell to the ground, pulling the table and all my textbooks and notes down on me. At the time, a sweeping sense of embarrassment ran through me and I jumped to my feet quickly, a nice shade of beetroot. I quickly exited the library.

Over the next few weeks, my breathing was very laboured, and climbing stairs between lectures and tutorials was a very arduous task. However, I assumed this was just a symptom of my CF. Then I felt a gurgling, bubble-like sensation when I was lying down. I went to my doctor in Blackrock Clinic for a check-up. Nothing came of it. The doctor advised me that if it continued, I was to call back in the week, so I continued in this discomfort.

A week later and my situation showed no improvement. Again I returned to Blackrock Clinic. This time, I was told I had a collapsed lung and I was rushed via ambulance to Mount Carmel Hospital for treatment. The doctor gave me a local anaesthetic. Within moments he was making an incision into my left side of my chest before the anaesthetic had kicked in, placing plastic tubing into the troubled area with considerable force, so much so that by the third push I screamed in agony. The doctor told me after he had completed the procedure that the pain felt was the equivalent of being shot. The tubing was then connected to plastic container to drain the lung of excess fluid. The procedure was not a success. I was now being scheduled for surgery on the Friday to 'reinflate' my lung. On the morning of the operation, I was prepared for surgery – kitted out in that flimsy, ass-exposing surgery gown and given the pre-med. A hazy daze engulfed me. After the procedure the physios would have to re-educate me as to how to breathe again.

Then the strangest thing happened. The surgery was postponed until the Monday due to a lack of surgical nurses. In

between that time, my father had been in consult?
American homoeopath called Vega Rosenberg an
about my current situation. I had previously
Mr Rosenberg on two occasions regarding co.. ⌐
support for cystic fibrosis, so he had knowledge of my case.
took my 'drug picture' – to borrow the homoeopathic term – and
he prescribed Carbo veg. Carbo veg is a remedy that 'has saved
many lives'.[7] Employing the knowledge of the 'Law of Similars',
the symptoms of Carbo veg at their most extreme are complete
state of collapse due to oxygen starvation, used in conjunction
with other efforts to revive respiration – most appropriate for my
current respiratory challenged state. Come the time for surgery
on Monday, I reported no pain or discomfort and X-rays showed
that my lung had 'reinflated'. I was discharged the following
morning. The energetic principles of homoeopathy saved me
going under the knife as the vibrational energetic qualities
'frequency matched' my symptoms and brought about a cure for
my collapsed lung. This was my first experience of the power and
subtlety of energy medicine, and it sowed the seed for exploring
such means for my health in the future.

Complex Homoeopathy

Complex homoeopathy is a combination of homoeopathics
synergistically employed to restore health. Our lifestyles have
changed considerably since Hahnemann's time. Our degraded
environment, poor diet and intake of prescription drugs leaves
our systems overworked, with little support in place to help.

New Vistas is a Limerick-based company that is leading the
way in complex homoeopathy. New Vistas products are designed
with a philosophy as well as a technology in place that is aware of
the challenges facing members of the public who want to remain
healthy through preventative means. Their programme for the
chronically ill addresses all stages in the restoration of balance.
Xenobiotics are an essential aid in the detoxification of foreign
chemicals from our bodies. Liquescences support and nourish
stressed or damaged organs. Sarcodes rebuild damaged organs and

---

[7] Helios, *Basic Guide to Homeopathy*

reatment remedies stimulate the body's own healing power. All provide essential minerals, vitamins and other ingredients to assist the body in functioning.

Through my search for complementary treatments to use as a support to conventional medicines, I have benefited greatly from complex homeopathics. The combination ingredients are based on a symptomatic picture and the combinations are developed to give a broadly based range of effectiveness. They are extremely safe to use, very effective and fast acting – as they are in liquid form, they are absorbed into the body more quickly.

The remedies I use are:

- XENOBIOTICS: as mentioned above, to stimulate the vital force within the body to cleanse itself and detoxify.

- BAC: a great means of treating bacterial infection.

- VIR: again, successful in the treatment of viral infection.

- LIQUESCENCES: as mentioned above, help to rebuild and strengthen the organ, enabling it to function as nature intended and restoring health to stressed organs.

- LUNG LIQUESCENCE: a nutritional remedy to support lung function.

- DIGESTIVE ENZYME LIQUESCENCE: stimulates the digestive enzyme release.

- MAGNESIUM LIQUESCENCE: promotes magnesium absorption and healthy body function. Magnesium is a natural broncodilator and, in liquid form, is the best means to absorb minerals.

- COLD LIQUESCENCE: prevention and treatment of the common cold. An excellent remedy for kicking a cold quickly. Taking this remedy every ten minutes for two hours before bed and the next morning, the symptoms and cold-like feeling will be greatly reduced.

Meridians: the Highway to Heaven

For centuries, using electromagnetic fields for healing was common practice. The Chinese, Indian and Tibetan cultures have described a surrounding substance of subtle energies that support, shape and animate the physical body. Each energy matrix they refer to is the same but labelled differently in each culture. The Chinese call it Ch'i, the Indians and Tibetans refer to it as Prana and in Japan it is called Ki. These 'subtle' energetic systems coordinate the life force with the body.

The meridians are the system of energy that the Chinese employ to restore Ch'i – an invisible nutritive energy that enters the body via the meridian points and brings life-giving nourishment to each organ. Meridians affect every organ and physiological system. There are fourteen meridian lines, twelve of them related to internal organs in the body: spleen, heart, small intestine, large intestine, bladder, kidney, circulation-sex, triple warmer,[8] gall bladder, lung, liver and stomach. Two are environmentally related – the central and governing meridians.

The Western world of medicine has only looked myopically at the meridian points, favouring more anatomically familiar models. However, meridian points have been utilised in the treatment of pain or for surgical anaesthesia in the Western world, but it is a very limited use indeed, considering the information that the meridians provide for the developing cells in the body. Many experiments have been done to prove the existence of a system of fine duct-like tubules that follow the descriptions of the ancient meridian pathways. Professor Kim Bong Han in Korea carried out experiments showing the anatomical nature of the meridian system in animals during the 1960s. He experimented on rabbits by injecting radioactive isotopes into their acupoint system and followed the uptake of the isotopes in the surrounding tissue. The technique used was microautoradiography, and it again showed the fine duct-like tubules that followed the meridian pathways. In further experimentation after proving the presence of the meridian pathways, he wished to confirm their

---

[8] The circulation-sex meridian has to do with the nutrition of new cells and the preparation for cell production (involving the menstrual cycle, ovarian and uterine functions, prostate and testicular functions). It also has to do with the handing down of genetic, cultural and personal heritage. The triple warmer meridian transfers information to all the meridians in the body and the organs they serve. It is the three 'heats' in the body – the heat of metabolism, maintaining body heat and the heat of 'fight or flight' or 'life passions'.

importance to the health of the organ's state. With knowledge of the pathways' energy-giving properties, he severed the line of energy to the liver in a frog. Shortly after severing the liver meridian, serious vascular degeneration took place throughout the whole liver. Repeated experimentation in this manner confirmed these results, concluding that energy flows from the meridian pathway to its respective organ, providing nutritional nourishment and appearing to interconnect with all cells/nuclei of the tissues.

A blockage in the line of these energy pathways results in a diseased organ, as is seen in Kim Bong Han's experiments. So, through a healthy flowing stream of energy, the meridians bring health and vitality to the body, remove blockages and determine the speed and form of cellular change. Their flow is as critical as the flow of blood; your life and health depend on both. 'If a meridian's energy is obstructed or unregulated, the system it feeds is jeopardised.'[9]

Employing the use of meridian pathways in our health consciousness would help us in the prevention of disease, for the physical body is the densest body of all and illness expresses itself physically last. Through understanding that illness is caused by energy imbalances within the meridians, we can see that the meridian changes mirror a dysfunction that has already occurred at the etheric level, and that these changes eventually filter down to the physical body via the meridian system. Meridian energy systems must be looked at and utilised more than the current myopic employment. The experiments of Professor Kim have clearly shown the intrinsic importance of meridians and the affect of imbalances in the meridian to the nuclei of cells.

Chakras – The Wheels of Life

Each chakra is a vortex of swirling energies impacting the organs, muscles, ligaments, veins and all other energy systems within its field.

> The soul is the holder of our life force energy, and this energy is further held together by our chakras. The soul works coopera-

---

[9] Eden and Feinstein, *Energy Medicine*, p.97

tively with our body, through the nervous system and brain, by managing the energy currents that provide us with life. Chakras receive the vital life force energy and distribute it to our total human energy field, as well as parts of the body nearest each chakra. This distribution of energy affects our mental and emotional behaviours. The energy or source of life, taken by the chakras, is known as prana or ch'i. We receive prana through proper breathing and air intake. When we receive a full, rich supply of ch'i energy, the chakras radiate intense bright colours. Simultaneously, the surrounding organs also receive full energy supplies and experience balance. When a chakra is not working properly or when there is an insufficient supply of ch'i energy, the chakra becomes weak, the immune system is depressed and disease or emotional instability.[10]

Seven major chakras exist in the body, from the base of your spine to the top of your head. Each chakra as mentioned is a power source of energy, providing lifeblood to the organs in proximity to the chakra.

From a physiological standpoint, the chakras appear to be involved in the flow of higher energies via a specific subtle energetic channels into the cellular structure of the physical body. At one level, they seem to function as energy transformers, stepping down energy of one form and frequency to a lower level energy. This energy is, in turn, translated into hormonal, physiological and ultimately cellular changes throughout the body.[11]

Dr Gerber's interpretation of the energy of chakras and Milanovich and McCune's accounts are very similar. Both expel the surrounding subtle energies between the etheric and physical bodies.

A balanced system is very important. A healthy, radiating chakra brings harmony and health to its holder, as well as emotional stability. I've found that much of the imbalance in life can be sourced to our chakras. Inability to speak up or incessant talking is a sign of a lack of harmony in the throat chakra, for example.

---

[10] McCune and Milanovich, *The Light Shall Set You Free*, p.87
[11] Gerber, *Vibrational Medicine*, p.128

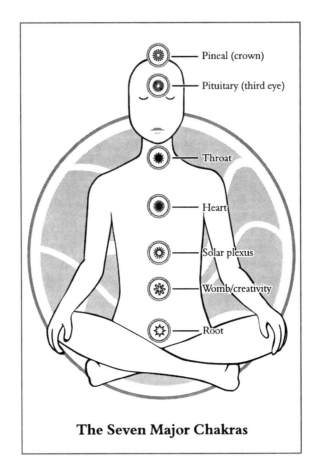

Pineal (crown)

Pituitary (third eye)

Throat

Heart

Solar plexus

Womb/creativity

Root

The Seven Major Chakras

AN OVERVIEW OF THE CHAKRA SYSTEM

- THE ROOT CHAKRA: located at the base of the spine, the root or base chakra is a receiver for Earth's subtle energies, literally grounding us. This chakra is primarily linked with survival. The need to support and protect family, eat and acquire are all governed by the root chakra. A balanced root chakra provides harmony and balance to these areas of your life. The chakra is red in colour and acts like all chakras – an energy transformer to the kidneys, adrenals and other organs along the spinal column.

- THE SACRAL CHAKRA: located a hand's width below the navel, the sacral chakra is the creative and imaginative force of the body. It is the birthplace of ideas and projects, embracing the creative flow that is within all of us. Think of its location – all the organs surrounding the sacral chakra are involved in creating a baby. When this chakra is in harmony, you are a confident, creative being that brings freedom, desire and pleasure into your life. The chakra is orange in colour and provides energies to the bladder, prostate, pancreas, genitals and reproductive organs.

- THE SOLAR PLEXUS: located a hand's width above the navel, the solar plexus is about individual identity. 'Your personal ego – your sense of who you are and who you are not – is forged within these energies: "this is who I am; this is who I want to be; this is how I want to be seen".'[12] It is often referred to as the *power* chakra. Too often we give our power away and it literally eats us up. Through a balanced solar plexus, people, emotions and situations have *'no power over you unless you give the power to them'*.[13] This chakra is yellow in colour and it is connected with the spleen, liver, gallbladder and stomach.

- THE HEART CHAKRA: located in the centre of your chest, the heart chakra is the emotional epicentre of our body, governing emotions such as joy, compassion, empathy, generosity and love. It is becoming the love that we are. A balanced heart chakra is one that forgives and lets go of negative energies that don't serve you, allowing you heal and change. The chakra is an emerald green colour and provides energy to the heart, lungs, circulatory system and thymus.

---

[12] Eden and Feinstein, *Energy Medicine*, p.152
[13] McCune and Milanovich, *The Light Shall Set You Free*, p.152

- THE THROAT CHAKRA: located in the throat, the throat chakra is all about expression and the ability to communicate clearly and truthfully. A balanced throat chakra gives you freedom to express what you mean and mean what you say. The chakra is aqua blue in colour and supplies energies to the vocal chords, voice and thyroid.

- THE THIRD EYE: located between the eyes, the third eye is the centre of wisdom in your body. It is where you get direction from within. A balanced third-eye chakra brings inner calm with self, the ability to clearly think out problems and find solutions, and the ability to have very strong connections with psychic power. The chakra is indigo in colour and transforms outer energies to support the pituitary gland and eyes.

- THE CROWN CHAKRA: located at the top of your head, the crown chakra is your connection to the life force of the universe; it is your divine energy. A balanced crown chakra is 'freedom from everything and union with all'.[14] Your crown chakra is the culmination of all other chakras and, being in harmony, raises your awareness and connection with the divine. The crown chakra is violet in colour and is a transformer of energy for the brain, the pineal gland and the whole body.

CHAKRA BALANCING EXERCISE

'Your awareness of your chakras is a prerequisite for a successful and meaningful meditation,' said Leni Morrison, Reiki Master and daughter of the Casa. A simple meditation I do is simply to find a quiet space for five minutes each day and sit in solitude.

- Beginning with a prayer of thanks, I slowly breathe in and out through my nose. Slowing down the breathing slows down the thought. I focus my energies and attention between my eyebrows and relax every part of my body.

- I breathe in love and light into my body and breathe out unwanted energies that do not serve my higher self.

---

[14] Dolores O'Reilly, *Chakra Therapy Course, Level One Manual*

- Focusing your energies on the chakras, start with the root chakra. Visualise a rich, red energy entering into your body with each breath, coursing down toward the base of your spine, and filling the base of your chakra with red energies that grow and glow with vibrancy. See that the energy cleanses the chakra of unwanted energies and restores harmony and balance to the base chakra, helping you ground with Mother Earth's energies.

- Moving to the sacral chakra, visualise a zesty orange energy entering into your body through the breath, coursing down toward the sacral chakra and filling it with orange energies that grow and glow with vibrancy. See that the energy cleanses the chakra of unwanted energies and restores harmony and balance, helping you embrace your creative being.

- Moving to the solar plexus, see the sunshine-yellow energy entering into your body through the breath coursing down, filling the chakra with yellow energies that grow and glow with vibrancy. See that the energy cleanses the chakra of unwanted energies and restores harmony and balance to the chakra, helping you step into and reclaim your power.

- Moving to the heart chakra, see the emerald-green energy entering into your body through the breath coursing down, filling the chakra with emerald-green energies that grow and glow with vibrancy. See that the energy cleanses the chakra of unwanted energies and restores harmony and balance, helping you become the love that you are and surrendering to the healing power of unconditional love. Now see that emerald green light transform energies in the heart.

- Moving up to the throat chakra, see the aqua blue energy entering into your body through the breath coursing down, filling the chakra with aqua blue energies that grow and glow with vibrancy. See that the energy cleanses the chakra of unwanted energies and restores harmony and balance, helping you communicate clearly and truthfully.

- Moving up to the third-eye chakra, see the indigo blue energy entering into your body through the breath coursing upwards and filling the chakra with indigo blue energies that grow and glow with vibrancy. See that the energy cleanses the chakra of unwanted energies and restores harmony and balance, helping you connect with your inner wisdom and intuition.

- Moving up to the final chakra – the crown chakra – visualise a violet energy entering into your body through the breath coursing upwards and filling the chakra with violet energies that grow and glow with vibrancy. See that the energy cleanses the chakra of unwanted energies and restores harmony and balance, helping you connect with your higher self.

- Sitting still in this beautiful energy, allow all of the colours to raise your vibration, heal you and lift your spirits. Now visualise all the chakra colours uniting in a beautiful spectrum of rainbow light, forming a united stream of white light connecting you with the divine, sending all the healing energies of the divine into your being via the chakras and sending that healing energy to all the organs in the proximity of each chakra.

Stay in this energy as long as feels comfortable and, when you wish to finish, work your way back down the chakras from the crown to the root chakra, asking that each chakra is in harmony and is safely cocooned in a protective white light.

Magnetostimulation

The healing potential of extremely low frequencies of magnetic fields (LFMF) in a wide variety of ailments has generated countless studies. Not to be confused with magnet therapy, a therapy with little or no scientific evidence, magnetostimulation is a revolutionary EU-certified medical apparatus in the treatment of physiological, neurological and psychological ailments.

Over the past fifteen years, research conducted in Poland by Professors Jaroszyk, Paluszak and Sieron (JPS) – the world's leading scientific experts in magnetostimulation – indicated that what was required for greater efficacy was not necessarily a higher level of magnetotherapy, but rather a weaker level, called magnetostimulation, which mimicked the body's own level. Using advanced computer technology, they were able to mix the patterns that allowed specific healing to take place at low strengths.

Following years of development research and testing, using a technology years ahead of competitors, they devised a product that would deliver the lower strength field that was required. The result of all this work was the introduction of the first Viofor JPS product into the European market in 2000.

Thousands of people in Europe have benefited from the use of the Viofor JPS System that is now widely used in Germany and France – as well as in its country of origin. In all these countries, it has been incorporated into conventional medical treatment and can now be found in hospitals, clinics and sports academies – as well as in patients' homes. Doctors in Europe agree that this is a remarkable system which combined with traditional treatments, will change the future of remedial therapy.

The generation of variable magnetic fields of extremely low frequencies and low intensity is well documented to have the following effects:

- analgesic
- anti-inflammatory
- anti-spastic
- regenerative

As a result, the Viofor JPS System helps the body return to its natural state of balance; this, in turn, leads to improved health and the reduction or elimination of many ailments. With its significant analgesic and regenerative effects on the body, it constitutes an excellent supplementary treatment, frequently enabling patients to decrease their usage of painkillers.

I used a Viofor JPS model with a view to improving my health. The use of extremely low frequencies resonated with me after all my reading and with the knowledge that we are all beings of vibration. Frequency matching my own innate healing patterns through a gentle non-invasive stimulation was a process I wanted to know more about and employ for my health. Using the Viofor JPS in respiration difficulties brings about an increase in the ciliary activity, helping to clean the lungs and expel the accumulated fluid. It was found to increase breathing effectiveness and decreased the number of episodes that lead to the scarring of the lungs in bronchiectasis.

The inactivity of a cystic fibrosis patient's sodium pump means that they have difficulty moving salt in and out of the cells. Mark Elkins, a researcher at Sydney's Royal Prince Alfred Hospital claims that scientists have long known about the importance of salt in understanding cystic fibrosis. Cystic fibrosis affects about 30,000 Americans. In a CF sufferer, the amount of salt and water that line the lungs' airways is not properly controlled, leading to a build-up of mucus. This blocks the airways and allows bacteria to breed. The problem is caused by a genetic defect.[15]

Magnetostimulation through the employment of Ionic Cyclotron Resonance is responsible for moving fluid in the body. It directly affects ions in the body, the most important being sodium. The intracellular processes are positively changed and homeostasis is improved, assisting the sodium pump efficiency by up to 30% after treatment.

★

Energy medicine and the Einstein formula have grown slowly in the medical fields. The biggest obstacle faced by energy medicine is the inability of science to define or measure energy.

> Whatever you cannot calculate you do not think is real. Since we cannot actually see energy, but only its outward manifestation, its origins may well lie in a reality beyond our senses.[16]

---

[15] See: Liz Szabo, 'Saltwater Therapy Helps Ease Cystic Fibrosis', *USA Today*, 18 January 2006
[16] Goethe quoted in: Callum Coats, *Living Energies*, p.36

Technology (Kirlian photography, EEG, EKG, etc.) has slowly come about to measure these subtle electromagnetic energetic fields, but the means are only giving a fragmented understanding of the wonder of the body's own energetic fields. The knowledge gained so far from these technologies has shown a correlation between a disruption in the energy patterns of the body and illness. As our technology evolves and becomes more sophisticated to include realms outside the physical body, the understanding gained about these energies will lead to a very exciting future.

NUTRITIONAL THERAPY
Healing with Foods

Let medicine be your food.

Hippocrates

Before the advent of pharmacologic drug therapy or surgery, doctors used the healing medicinal qualities of food to restore health to the sufferer. Nutrition embraces the philosophies of the famous Greek doctor and founder of Western medicine, Hippocrates, to help people of all ages to stay at their personal peak of energy and vitality. He promoted the healing energies of medicinal herbs, spices and food as the primary tools for healing, and if they did not assist then the route of drug therapy and surgery would follow. Today, medicine bypasses nutrition as a preventative medicine and goes straight to chemically treating the patient. In fact, medical students today have only seven hours over six years of medical schooling dedicated to the role of nutrition in healing.

With a growing body of work studying the medicinal healing qualities of food, it is surprising that the notion of healing through eating is not being adequately taken into account by the medical profession. If food is our medicine and medicine is our food, then let food be our tool for healing. The frenetic pace at which we lead our lives and our improper nutrition affect the experience, purpose and pleasure of food. Dashboard dining is becoming paramount as we are stuck in congested traffic or rushing to and from work. The widespread use of microwaves does not take into consideration the harmful electromagnetic affect it has on foods – transforming the amino acid from L-proline to D-proline, a proven toxin to the nervous system, liver and kidneys. Lifestyle and nutrition are clearly linked. The return of farmers' markets throughout Ireland, for example, shows that consumer confidence is growing disillusioned with the quality of supermarket microwave meals and tinned processed foods, and returning to home-grown, local produce. The consumers are voting with their feet.

With the return of farmers' markets, we are returning to nature. We had community-based living prior to chemical farming. Agriculture and man worked in harmony, producing for the local community, not for the needs of giant food conglomerates. In the 1940s, chemical farming became commonplace. It adopted the principles of the German chemist, Baron Justus von Liebig, who carried out many studies looking into elements and chemicals required by plants for growth, no doubt in a sincere effort to rectify soil deficiencies and increase fertility. The result of the von Liebig studies was the employment of nitrogen, potassium and phosphorous – or NPK. Though this was a very simple employment by the chemical manufacturers, von Liebig later admitted that the requirement for chemically healthy soil was more complex than the simple use of NPK. The outcome of pumping the soil with harmful chemicals has reduced the soil to a lifeless mass and depleted its fertility. As Schauberger so crudely put it:

> Contemporary agriculture treats Mother Earth like a whore and rapes her. All year round it scrapes away her skin and poisons it with artificial fertiliser, for which a science is to be thanked that has lost all connection with nature.[17]

Nutritional Therapy

> Nature produces no diseases, nor deformities.
>
> George Catlin

A monk asks, 'Is there anything more miraculous than the wonders of nature?' I say, 'Yes – your appreciation of the wonders of nature.' Viktor Schauberger substantiates this with his formula of $N = C^2$, which means that to work with the laws of nature, you

---

[17] From the Schauberger Archives. See Coats, *Living Energies*, p.261

must first comprehend nature, then copy nature. Too often, man has flexed his muscle to better nature – e.g. in the shift away from local produce that works with the seasons to chemical agriculture, as mentioned above. Prior to that, agriculture had been carried out on nature's terms with man cooperating with the land. Today we have farmers who produce technological food based on the latest discoveries as to how our vegetation and plant life should grow and behave. This microcosm is the antithesis of the macrocosm of natures' kingdom.

Nutritional therapy looks at illness though the eyes of nature, and corrects the wrongs of industry/lifestyles with the rights of nature. Patricia Quinn writes about the 'The Four Doctors':[18]

1. sunlight and fresh air

2. proper exercise and sufficient rest

3. good food

4. pure water

1. SUNLIGHT AND FRESH AIR

All of the above are basic and intrinsic requirements for good health. Solar energy from sunlight will provide you with vitamin D. Fresh air is necessary so our bodies can exchange toxins and pollutants in our systems for good, clean air. However, the quality of our fresh air is being harmed through the noxious fumes and vapours of industry and motor vehicles. The increase in industry, the methods used for energy generation and deforestation disrupt the natural conditions for creating and maintaining health. The natural temperature of our environment is raised, 'thus bringing about subtle and sometimes lethal changes in cellular function. In other words the anomaly state of health...'[19]

A study conducted at Lancaster University in England under the direction of Dr John Whitelegg looked at the health of over 1,000 households fronting major traffic arteries. The study showed a clear correlation between respiratory disease and traffic

[18] Patricia Quinn, *Healing with Nutritional Therapy*, Newleaf, UK, 1998, p.5

[19] Coats, *Living Energies*, p.105

fumes. It was also found that people near such congested areas were more susceptible to disease and that headaches, itchy eyes and general fatigue were commonplace.

2. PROPER EXERCISE AND SUFFICIENT REST

Office work, desk jobs and a different pace of life to our ancestors is playing a role in our current state of health. This lifestyle is not what our bodies are designed for, and our physiology has not yet transformed to adapt to this abnormal use of the human body. The body needs movement and activity to maintain normal functions. If the body functions normally, it will know when to eat and in what quantity. Combined with overeating, lack of sufficient exercise puts our body's functions under extra pressure to break down excess fats that accumulate due to our inactivity. Exercise is important to maintain a healthy immune system and release stress. It gives the body more energy and builds up strength.

Rest is also an important factor, allowing the body to catch up on itself. With all the constant stresses and pressures of daily living, it is important to help the body cleanse and regenerate. Inability to let the body catch up and self-cleanse, and a constant go-go-go attitude leads to a fight-and-flight mentality that is usually self-induced, leaving the body depleted and open to illness such as infection, immune system weakness, lymphatic congestion and so on. Let go and relax!

3. GOOD FOOD

Moving onto the benefits of good food, the ability of herbs and spices to heal has been documented for centuries, dating as far back as Ancient Greece, from Asklepios to Hippocrates (400 BC) and following on to Roman times (first century AD). Food was the medicine of the day, utilising the healing properties of herbs to remedy an ailment, and employing to totality the benefits of the plant rather than finding an active substance as favoured by science. Take foxglove, for instance. It has been used throughout the ages as a means to successfully treat illnesses, ranging from fluid retention to heart difficulties. Modern science has isolated the active substance – digitalis – as the healing property, thus ignoring the synergistic elements of foxglove.

Nutritional therapy is a 'system of healing based on the belief that food as nature intended provides medicine we need to obtain and maintain a state of health'.[20] The maxim 'we are what we eat' is very true when we fill our bodies with microwave meals, takeaways and sugary, processed foods. They all provide little nutritional quality and greatly give rise to illness. Our foods are playing a key role in the state of our health. Today, headaches affect over 20% of the civilised population. In the 1930s, Dr Weston Price conducted an interesting study of traditional groups and their change to a more processed Westernised diet. When the Gaelic people, living in the Hebrides off the coast of Scotland, changed from their traditional diet of small seafoods and oatmeal to modernised diet of 'angel food cake, white bread and many white flour commodities, marmalade, canned vegetables, sweetened fruit juices, jams and confections', first generation children became mouth-breathers and their immunity to the diseases of civilisation reduced dramatically. The traditional diet of the Hebrides Gaelic people was found to be four times the nutritional quality of the modern diet counterpart.[21]

Nutritional therapy is more important than ever with Westernised industrial foods being the staple diet of our world. These harmful foods go against the laws of nature and reap a bitter harvest of man-made diseases. The quality of our foods has changed drastically over the last 100 years – more than over the last 100,000. High fat, high salt and high sugar products are primary factors in our daily dining experience.

> A diet in which a high proportion of the energy content comes from refined sugars (sugary snacks, drinks and confectionery) tends to be low in vitamins, minerals and dietary fibre. Consumption of refined sugars in Europe and the United States now supplies an average of 14–17% of energy, with some children consuming even higher amounts of around 17–20%.[22]

---

[20] Quinn, *Healing with Nutritional Therapy*, p.1

[21] See: Dr Andrew Weston Price, *Nutrition and Physical Degeneration*, Keats Publications, 15th Edition, 2003

[22] Michael van Straten, *The Healthy Food Directory*, Newleaf, UK, 1999, p.196

Refined sugars affect the adrenal system (the body's natural steroid), rob us of our B-vitamins and cause our all-important bone-building minerals to start to leak out from their storage sites. Breakfast is the most important meal of the day. It is literally 'breaking your fast' and it ends the longest time that our bodies go without food. What we consume at breakfast is key to the kind of energy we want for the rest of the day. Substituting your consumption of sugary, processed, glossy, marketable breakfast cereals for a breakfast such as porridge is one great way to provide the body with a slow releasing natural energy. It provides fibre, energy and contains no addictives, colours or preservatives. I add some dried fruit and honey to my porridge and sprinkle on half a teaspoon of Vidacell (see below) and it keeps me energised until lunch.

The nutritional quality of white bread is minute to say the least. Again, in Dr Price's book, *Nutrition and Physical Degeneration*, he shows the nutritional quality of white flour was sacrificed for shipping reasons and to prevent insect infestation. The flour contained was four-fifths phosphorous and had nearly all nutrients and vitamins removed during the processing stage. 'Tests showed that white bread was unable to sustain insect life, while half a slice of whole rye bread was totally consumed by bugs.'[23]

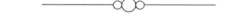

VIDACELL: A CELLULAR FUNCTIONAL FOOD

Fifteen years of research… thousands of years of Mother Nature.

Vidacell is a unique functional food that helps reverse the cellular aging process by providing the essential nutrients necessary to protect, repair and renew the body at a cellular level. Vidacell's all natural proprietary formulation promotes cellular energy

---

[23] Price, *Nutrition and Physical Degeneration*

(ATP), which is essential fuel for the body. Vidacell contains a complete amino acid profile, complex carbohydrates and cofactors necessary for life, all in bio-available form for complete and immediate utilisation by the body.

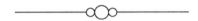

Eating Healing Foods

Eating leafy green vegetables and other seasonal fruit and vegetables is best for your health, particularly if they are chemical free and produced locally. Manufacturers of chemical sprays may point out that the quantity of food their products generate is greater, but the cost is continuously decreasing quality at the expense of life, as chemicals cause your breathing rate to increase as your body tries to clear the toxicity.

Eating the recommended daily five portions of fruit and vegetables is the starting point to a healthy diet. Important research documents the role of the antioxidants present in fruit and vegetables in preventing chronic diseases. Fruit is very important – full of vitamins, minerals, antioxidants and fibre – all vital for health. As far back as 1747, James Lind discovered that lemons and oranges helped to reverse the symptoms of scurvy. This showed the possibilities for vitamins and fruit being used as a medicine.

This has been further documented through numerous studies showing the healing qualities of foods. Apples and tomatoes are 'good for lungs' according to a study carried out by the British Thoracic Society under the direction of Dr John Harvey at Nottingham University.[24] Both tomatoes and apples are very rich in antioxidants and those antioxidants have a positive effect on lung function. Apples contain high levels of an antioxidant flavonoid called quercetin, and may be important in protecting the lungs from the harmful effects of the atmosphere and even cigarette smoke. 'The latest study confirms that regular intake of

[24] 'Apples and Tomatoes "Good for Lungs",
http://news.bbc.co.uk/1/hi/health/1343502.stm, 22 May 2001

fresh fruit reduces the risk of developing respiratory disease and represents a simple effective intervention that everyone can adopt to help keep themselves fit,' says Dr Martyn Partridge, Chief Medical Adviser for National Asthma Campaign. 'Apples are also a very good tonic for the heart and circulation as they are rich in a soluble fibre, pectin, which can help eliminate cholesterol and protects against environmental pollutants.'[25]

All fruit and vegetables have therapeutic properties that can assist the body in healing. Pears, for instance, contain the soluble fibre, pectin, which reduces cholesterol. Pears are also a valuable aid for regulating the bowels. Strawberries can help in the treatment of gout and arthritis as they help eliminate the joint-irritating uric acid from the body, and they can also reduce blood pressure. Consequently, they are recommended as a therapeutic aid in the alleviation of kidney stones. Blackcurrants help in the prevention and treatment of food poisoning due to their antibacterial effect. Leafy green vegetables such as cabbage, broccoli, kale and kelp are very good as they are excellent sources of magnesium and calcium. Turnip greens, for example, provide twice as much calcium as milk and can be an important calcium substitute for people who are lactose intolerant. These are just some of a host of healing fruit and vegetables that can act as a natural remedy for the body.

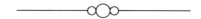

JUICING

A great way that I've found for getting my five portions of fruit and vegetables per day is through
juicing. Liquids offer a quick way to absorb all my
vitamins and minerals. Though nature designed our
system to break down and absorb all the nutrients
from our foods, the system is and has been under
pressure due to our poor diets and stressed,
overworked organs.

---

[25] Ibid.

> [Juicing does] the work that your body normally has
> to. It takes whole fruits and veg and miraculously
> extracts the pure liquid gold that is so easy for the
> body to digest and assimilate.[26]

Therefore, juicing allows the cells in the body to receive the full benefit of the fruit's healing potential, as opposed to if it were to process the fruits itself. A little side tip would be the edition of Udo's oil, which contains the essential fatty acids (omega-3, 6 and 9) that the body cannot produce, and is an excellent immune-system booster and energy provider. The combinations of the fruit offset the taste. Adding cranberry juice to the mix is also very beneficial, as a glass of cranberry juice a day is ten times more effective at killing urinary bacteria than conventional medicines and sufferers can stay infection free if a glass a day is upheld.

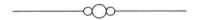

The Future of Nutrition: *Nutrigenomics*

Though still in embryonic stages, nutrigenomics is an area of great excitement and potential. The central premise is 'personalised nutrition' and 'promises to improve health conditions and to prevent disease e.g. diabetes, obesity, cardiovascular diseases and cancer. On the basis of results from nutrigenomics research, new types of functional foods with proven health claims could be developed, and perhaps personalised diets created – based on an individual's genetic make-up.'[27]

It is a science that looks at an individual's reaction to food compounds and measures how what we eat interacts with our bodies. The overall goal is to understand how the whole body

---

[26] Jason Vale, *The Juice Master's Ultimate Fast Food: Discover the Power of Raw Juice*, Thorsons, UK, 2003, p.43

[27] See: *www.nugo.org*

(genes, proteins and metabolism) responds to foods. Professor Mike Gibney of Trinity College Dublin is leading the field of nutrigenomics in Ireland and the EU. At the Flora Institute conference on nutrigenomics, he commented:

> Nutritionists are beginning to examine the variation that occurs between people in their genetic code. These tiny differences on the genome lead to small but significant changes in how nutrients are metabolised in the body. In terms of heart health, people may differ in how their cholesterol levels will respond to changes in fat type or content some may need more folic acid than others.[28]

This knowledge could then be used as a preventative means for people who may have a genetic predisposition to illness, thus coming full circle to Hippocrates' guiding principal in 400 BC: 'let food be thy medicine'.

4. GOOD WATER

> All is born of water and upheld by water too!

> Goethe

For your system to function, the role of water is vital in metabolism, assimilation, the regulation of body temperature and the nourishment of the body. The performance of our bodily functions will not be effective without the correct levels of water in our body. Today our systems are chronically dehydrated, and a dehydrated body is a disease producer. Medicine's chemical products silence the signals, thus ignoring our body's cry for water.

> The various signals produced by these water distributors are indicators of regional thirst and drought of the body. At the onset, they can be relieved by an increased intake of water, yet they are improperly dealt with by the use of commercial chemical products until pathology is established and diseases are born.[29]

---

[28] From: *The Irish Pharmacist,* Vol. 7, Issue 6, June 2005
[29] Dr F Batmanghelidj, *Your Body's Many Cries for Water: A Revolutionary Natural Way to Prevent Illness and Restore Good Health*, Tagman Press, UK, 2000, p.10

Our metabolism and assimilation becomes sluggish as a result of mixed signals between thirst and hunger. The brain signals the need for energy. Hydroelectricity as an energy provider for the body is more urgent than energy from sugar in the bloodstream. However, both hunger and thirst signals are activated simultaneously with the majority of the public reaching for (sugary) snacks to counter this energy depletion, instead of water. This confusion causes eating when we should be drinking and affects our waistlines. As only 20% of energy via sugar in the bloodstream reaches the brain, the rest is absorbed into our body and, due to our inactive lifestyles, it stays on our waistline. Water and its hydroelectric energy-giving properties provides the body with the needed energy, and any excess energy the body does not burn is passed out in the form urine from the body.

The intake of water is key before all meals as it helps the digestion process. A healthy, hydrated cell membrane is a 'waterway' for enzyme activity (improving the digestive process).

When our body is the correct temperature (37 °C), we are healthy, vibrant beings. 'Good water is the preserver of our proper bodily temperature, our anomaly point of greatest health and energy...'[30]

Nourishment and healing for our bodies is provided in many ways by water: it provides the body with human fuel (hydroelectricity), lubrication for the joints (as the synovial fluid is primarily water based), and breathing is also assisted through hydrating the lungs with water to counter moisture loss, as much water is lost through perspiration. The healing ability of water as a preventative is applicable to a whole host of ailments. We now need water to take its mantle in modern medicine as the panacea to all ills, and recognise this elixir of life. 'The upholder of the cycles which support the whole of life is *water*. In every drop of water dwells a deity...'[31]

---

[30] Coats, *Living Energies*, p.113
[31] Viktor Schauberger, *Our Senseless Toil*, 1933

Now good digestion wait on appetite, and health on both!

William Shakespeare

Adhering to and using these principles as our guiding light can play a dynamic role in our health. The body is more than the sum of its parts, and feeding the body the essential elements of sunlight, air, food, water and exercising the system will ensure a healthy vital being. The synergistic employment of the 'Four Doctors' for healing is key to the future of health and the growing power of preventative rather than curative medicine.

EMOTIONAL FREEDOM TECHNIQUES

Tap into Health

What is hidden within will dictate what will appear on the outside.

El Morya

Emotions and their link to our physical well-being is gaining more and more credence with our health today. The conflict between psychological and somatic symptoms represents the fine line between our emotional states. 'As patients, we are perpetrator and victim rolled into one, constantly suffering from nothing more than our own unconsciousness.'[32] This condition manifests itself physically in some form or another if we are not adept or we do not wish to face an aspect of our character, confront a conflict or address an emotion, hence suppressing the unconscious state. The suppressed form manifests itself through the physical.

The efforts of modern medicine in addressing physical illness today have been through material means, as mentioned in the first chapter. Though successful in the short term, the success is down to temporary containment of the physical expression rather than cure. If the means by which the symptom has arisen are not addressed and treatment is continued, then the symptom will find another way to show itself.

Disease is, in essence, the result of conflict between soul and mind, and will never be eradicated except by spiritual and mental effort. Such efforts, if properly made with understanding, can cure and prevent disease by removing those basic factors which are its primary cause. No effort directed to the body alone can do more than superficially repair damage, and in this there is no

---

[32] Dahlke and Dethlefsen, *The Healing Power of Illness*, p.75

cure, since the cause is still operative and may again demonstrate its presence in another form.[33]

Our words, thoughts and actions all carry vibration. The vibrational power of these words, thoughts and actions can be the wedge between our body and soul if they carry a negative frequency. Our mouth can be personal enemy number one! The total oblivious nature and reckless disregard of our speech and thoughts has a great impact on our life and our emotions. We are responsible for many conditions of our lives and have the free will to change the nature of our lives and environment. In grasping the reins of our destiny, we must let our thoughts, words and actions be one, and realise that the energies we use – whether positive or negative – are the energies we send out and attract. Today, more than ever, we place such strong emphasis on our physical well-being and our health. Many of us are careful about the foods we ingest, limit the amount of alcohol we consume, know the importance of exercise and so on, but we put little time into our emotional health. Feeding our hearts and minds with healthy positive thoughts and using affirmations can have a profound healing effect on the body and the soul. Energy goes where attention flows, so direct your time and energies into creating a landscape of vitality.

Affirmations

One powerful way to shape and manifest our lives and environment is through the use of affirmations. Affirmations help us to gather our thoughts and focus our energies into supporting our needs and setting us up on the path to realise all we deserve.

> Therefore I say to you, whatever things you ask when you pray, believe that you receive them, and you will have them.
>
> Mark 11:24, King James Bible

The use of affirmations is a very self-empowering tool. All of us have a little 'inner chatterbox' that imprison us and limits our

---

[33] Bach, *Heal Thyself*, pp.2–3

potential through our negative nature or fear. This limiting brain drain paralyses us from realising our ability to 'self-actualise'. Using affirmations frees us from our own oppressive shackles and helps to us make real our needs, dreams and aspirations.

When writing an affirmation, make it simple, short and positive, always stating it in the now. I have employed several affirmations to the betterment of my health and lungs. Here are a few examples that I have borrowed or written:

- Every day, in every way, I feel better and better.

- My health and lungs are perfect and I am stronger every day.

- Now I can focus my mind on the present and not worry about other things. *Dr Bach*

- Now I can think good of myself and others. *Dr Bach*

- I can do all things through God, who strengthens me. *Vincent Norman Pearle*

- I am a vibrant being of light and my cells shine brightly in this light.

Emotional Freedom Techniques (EFT)[34]

Where astonishing emotional relief leads to profound healings.

THE QUEST

Gary Craig is a Stanford engineer who is the founding father of Emotional Freedom Techniques (or EFT), which have developed from the principles of Thought Field Therapy, developed by Dr Callahan. Years ago, he saw a direct correlation between one's emotional health and quality of life. In realising this, Mr Craig spent years consuming multitudes of textbooks on psychology, psychotherapy and neurolinguistic programming, attended a vast array of courses and talked with many practitioners in the field of

---

[34] See *www.emofree.com*

mental and emotional health to find the best means to ᵤ
healthy emotional state. Though the effectiveness of the ᵤ
fields cannot be questioned, his hunger for emotional well-be
and vitality with long-lasting results drove him to contin
looking beyond the conventional approaches. He wanted to find a
solution that could be applied to all negative emotions, with a
result that would free the person from their psychological
paralysis.

After years of searching, the answer arrived in the form of
'tapping' your fears, worries, phobias and all negative emotions
away. A Californian psychologist, Dr Callahan, was employing
a tapping technique that was giving immense relief from
intense negative emotions in minutes, and EFT developed
from here.

DR CALLAHAN'S DISCOVERY AND THE FOUNDING OF THOUGHT FIELD THERAPY

Dr Callahan's discovery was based on the Chinese knowledge of
meridians, as discussed earlier. Our bodies have a profound
electrical nature and our electrical systems are vital to our physical
well-being. Employing the system of energy circuits, meridians,
once stimulated through tapping, can have a profound effect on
physical and emotional health. These changes would not occur if
there was no energy system.

The proof of this lay in the employment of the technique.
After fruitless years of treating a patient who had an intense
phobia of water, Dr Callahan decided to move beyond psychotherapy and asked his client where the phobia felt strongest in the
body. On locating the emotional discomfort zone in the body, he
proceeded to tap under his client's eye (the meridian point of the
stomach that is associated with fears and phobias). Within
moments of correcting the energy imbalance, his client reported
instant calm and that the phobia was no longer there. His client
raced to the nearest swimming pool and felt no fear. The
paralysing, immobilising phobia had gone.

BATTERIES NOT INCLUDED... PSYCHOLOGICAL REVERSAL

The procedure of EFT is laid out in the following exercise. First, I would like to mention a little bit more about the set-up and Psychological Reversal (PR). The set-up is key to EFT. Once you have zoned in on the area you want worked on (be it fear, phobia, worry, physical pain, etc.) and written out your affirmation, the next step is to programme the affirmation into the body via the set-up. The set-up is the trigger point for correcting psychological reversal.

Throughout our lives, maintaining our emotional balance is very difficult. The stresses of work and the demands of life cause disharmony, which throws us out of our natural rhythm. The little things suddenly become huge and our ability to rationalise goes out of the window. It is a self-created, self-defeating, head-against-the-wall, frustrating, unproductive existence that we inhabit.

Psychological reversal is caused by 'negative thinking, which often occurs subconsciously and outside of your awareness'. Mr Craig uses an analogy of batteries with the wrong polarity. Consider a typical hand-held electronic device, such as a CD player. These devices require batteries in order to run. It is equally important that these batteries are installed properly. If the + and - signs are pointing in the wrong direction, the device will not work. The device is not broken, but if the batteries are not correctly aligned then the device will behave exactly as if there were no batteries in it at all. This analogy represents what we mentioned at the outset – the destructive nature of negative thinking on our emotional health. That 'ah, what is the point' mentality takes hold of the client. A self-defeated mentality is induced. For example, an overweight individual may not be overly motivated to shed the pounds for the simple thought that they will just end up spending money changing their wardrobe. Or consider the football striker who has lost his 'Midas touch' in front of the goal – he would definitely be suffering from psychological reversal. So how do we reset this self-destruct button?

The set-up part of the EFT exercise works by addressing the PR point, forming an affirmation as already mentioned and finally by rubbing or tapping the 'sore spot'.

To find your sore point, place your right hand on your collarbone and run your thumb and middle finger toward each other till they meet at the U-point of the collarbone. Then, run both your thumb and middle finger down an inch from the U-point and out an inch. Both finger and thumb should fall into a natural groove in your chest cavity or the point of soreness. It is sore as it is part of the lymphatic system. The reason for the lymphatic system being sore is that, unlike its fluid cousin, blood, the lymphatic system does not have the luxury of the heart to pump the lymphatic fluid around the body. The lymphatic system is exercised through movement, walking, swimming, running, etc. As long as there is movement the lymphatic system shall be in a healthy state. When you've located this point, tap or gently rub the point while saying aloud your positively stated affirmation three times. Alternatively, you can tap the side of your hand (the karate chop point) and the procedure will still work. I personally favour the point on the chest as it is also the K-27 point in kinesiology (a point for creating natural energy in the body as mentioned in the third chapter).

The set-up is the clearing factor of the exercise. As mentioned earlier, it is the memory recall stage and after that allows the energy imbalance to be addressed. Please see the following exercise for the remaining stages.

EFT Exercise

THE SET-UP

Start off by stimulating the sore spot (a natural little hollow in your chest around an inch below your collarbone) or tapping the side of hand while repeating an affirmation three times.

The affirmation: Even though I have this _____ I deeply and completely accept myself.

For example: Even though I have this *headache/fear of spiders/craving for sweets, etc.* I deeply and completely accept myself.

The purpose of an affirmation is acknowledging the problem and creating self-acceptance, despite the existence of the problem.

THE SEQUENCE

This stage involves tapping and stimulating each energy point seven times or more while repeating your affirmation to yourself.

The points to tap are the following:

- eyebrow (EB),
- side of eye (SE),
- under eye (UE),
- under nose (UN),
- chin (CH),
- collarbone (CB),
- underarm (UA),
- below nipple (BN),
- thumb (TH),
- index finger (IF),
- middle finger (MF),
- baby finger (BF),
- side of hand (SH).

THE 9 GAMUT POINT

The purpose of this point is to promote harmony between both spheres of the brain through eye movement, counting and humming. Through connecting nerves, certain parts of the brain are stimulated when the eyes are moved. We engage the right side of the brain when we creatively hum a tune of some sort and the left rational side of brain is activated with the counting process of 1–5.

1. Close your eyes.

2. Open your eyes.

3. Look down to the right.

4. Look down to the left.

5. Roll your eyes in a clockwise direction.

6. Roll your eyes in a counter-clockwise movement.

7. Hum a tune aloud for two seconds (my favourite is Madonna's 'Like a Virgin', but any humtastic tune will do).

8. Count rapidly from 1–5.

9. Finish off by humming your song again.

The Tapping Points and the Associated Meridians

TAPPING POINT	ORGAN	EMOTION
EB	Bladder	Trauma, frustration, restlessness
SE	Gall bladder	Rage
UE	Stomach	Anxiety, fear, cravings, phobias, nerves
UN	Governing vessel	Embarrassment, psychological reversal
CH	Central vessel	Shame
CB	Kidney	Fear, anxiety, insecurity
UA	Spleen	Anxiety, cravings, self-esteem, nerves
BN	Liver	Anger, unhappiness
TH	Lung	Pride, intolerance, arrogance
IF	Large Intestine	Guilt and forgiveness
MF	Circulation sex	Broken heart, addictive cravings
BF	Heart	Anger, loss, self-forgiveness
SH	Psychological reversal	Sadness

This is the layout of the EFT Basic Recipe as per EFT Manual, sixth ed. The choice of theme tune to hum along to can be altered according to personal preference.

CONCLUSION

Only in the last three years have I started to see real bountiful benefits in my health. A key reason for writing this book is an important lesson I've learnt – the importance of taking command of your illness, whatever it may be, and stopping the abdication of control and responsibility to everyone else. Only then will you begin the power to heal.

Albert Schweitzer (1875–1965), doctor and philosopher, said, 'Within every patient there resides a doctor', and by tapping into this hidden healer and doctor within, an amazing paradigm shift occurs in our health. We no longer become pill-popping automatons, but can embrace instead the Bach philosophy of 'heal thyself'. The effect ripples like a stone skimmed across water, growing exponentially with each ripple.

BIBLIOGRAPHY

Bach, Dr Edward, *Heal Thyself: An Explanation of the Real Cause and Cure of Disease*, Random House UK, newly ed. edition, 2004

Batmanghelidj, Dr F, *Your Body's Many Cries for Water: A Revolutionary Natural Way to Prevent Illness and Restore Good Health*, Tagman Press, UK, 2000

Brundtland, Gro Harlem, *Our Common Future*, Oxford University Press, 1988

Butts, Robert F and Jane Roberts, *Seth Speaks: The Eternal Validity of the Soul*, Amber-Allen Publishing, USA, 1994

Catlin, George, *Shut Your Mouth and Save Your Life*, London, N Truebner and Co., 1870

Coats, Callum, *Living Energies: An Exposition of Concepts Related to the Theories of Viktor Schauberger*, Gateway, second edition, USA, 2002

Dahlke, Rudiger and Thorwald Dethlefsen, *The Healing Power of Illness: The Meaning of Symptoms and How to Interpret Them*, Element Books Limited, 1997

Eden, Donna and David Feinstein, *The Energy Medicine Kit*, Sounds True, Kit Edition, USA, 2005

——, *Energy Medicine: Balance your Body's Energies for Optimum Health, Joy and Vitality*, Penguin, SA, 2000

Gerber MD, Richard, *Vibrational Medicine: The #1 Handbook for Subtle-Energy Therapies*, Bear & Company, UK, 2001

Helios, *Basic Guide to Homeopathy*

Kazarinov, V A, 'The Biochemical Basis of K P Buteyko's Theory of Disease of Deep Respiration', in *Buteyko Method: Experience of Implementation in Medical Practice*, ed. by K P Buteyko, Moscow, Patriot Press, 1990

McCune, S D and N J Milanovich, *The Light Shall Set You Free*, Athena Publishing, 1996

McKeown, Patrick G, *Asthma Free Naturally: Everything You Need to Know About Taking Control of Your Asthma*, Harper Thorsons, London, 2005

Motluk, Alison, 'Curry spice could alleviate cystic fibrosis', *Newscientist.com* news service, 22 April 2004

O'Donohue, J, *Eternal Echoes: Celtic Reflections on our Yearning to Belong*, Bantam Press, 2000

O'Reilly, Dolores, *Chakra Therapy Course, Level One Manual*

Price, Dr Andrew Weston, *Nutrition and Physical Degeneration*, Keats Publications, fifteenth edition, 2003

Quinn, Patricia, *Healing with Nutritional Therapy*, Newleaf, UK, 1998

Siegel, B S, *Love, Medicine and Miracles*, Arrow Books, 1988

Sky, Michael, *Breathing: Expanding Your Power and Energy*, Bear & Company, UK, 1990

Szabo, Liz, 'Saltwater Therapy Helps Ease Cystic Fibrosis', *USA Today*, 18 January, 2006

Schauberger, Viktor, 'The Forest and its Significance (Der Wald und seine Bedeutung)', *Tau Magazine*, vol. 146

——, *Our Senseless Toil*, 1933

van Straten, Michael, *The Healthy Food Directory*, Newleaf, UK, 1999

Vale, Jason, *The Juice Master's Ultimate Fast Food: Discover the Power of Raw Juice*, Thorsons, UK, 2003

Websites

www.NewScientist.com

www.newvistashealthcare.com

www.greatlifeintl.com

www.nugo.org

www.emofree.com

RESOURCE GUIDE

Ireland

Energy medicine, homeopathy, NLP, electromagnetic stimulation, kinetic energy, thermal therapy, sound therapy:

Breda and Ed Morrison
Tuan Health Sanctuary
Castle Hill
Enniscorthy
Co. Wexford
Ireland
+353 53 92 35712

Sister Rachel Hoey
St Raphela's
Stillorgan
Co. Dublin
+353 1 2889559

Complex homeopathy:

Martin Murray
New Vistas
Plassey Park
Limerick
www.newvistashealthcare.com
+353 61 334455

Also check out Mr Murray's
new Dublin establishment:
Dublin Nutricentre
28 South William Street
Dublin 2
+353 1 6333535

Reiki:

Marilen Morrison
Tuan Health Sanctuary
Castle Hill
Enniscorthy
Co. Wexford
Ireland
+353 53 92 35712

Delores O'Reilly
Radhare Na dTonna
Ballynabarney
Wicklow PO
Co. Wicklow
+353 86 841 85 13

Nutrition:

Patricia Quinn
Sunnyhill
Bohernabreena
Dublin 24
+353 1 4513619
Please contact between the hours of 10 a.m.–2 p.m.

Buteyko Breathing:

Patrick McKeown
Buteyko Breathing
Administration and Galway Clinic
Unit 6
Calbro House
Tuam Road
Co. Galway
www.asthmacare.ie
Freephone: 1800 93 1935
Runs workshops around the
country.

Charles Maguire
The Buteyko Centre
Derryclogher
Borlin
Bantry
Co. Cork
www.thebuteykocentre.com
Phone: +353 27 66209

Ayurveda Medicine:

Dr Donn Brennan
Number 9
Longford Terrace
Monkstown
Dublin
+353 1 284 5742
www.ayurveda.ie

United Kingdom

Medicahealth Ltd., distributors to the Viofor JPS system and Theragem
technology
Dewhurst Road
Langho
Blackburn
BB6 8AF
UK
www.medicahealth.org
UK: +44 870 609 4583
Ireland: +353 53 9235712

The Sanctuary of Healing
Dewhurst Road
Langho
Blackburn
BB6 8AF
UK
www.thesanctuaryofhealing.co.uk
Tel: +44 125 424 6940

Tricia Courtney Dickens
Chi Machine Distributor
Down to Earth Holistic Health
209 Tangier Road
Baffins
Portsmouth
Hampshire
UK: +44 239 279 3720
Ireland: +353 53 92 35712

Society for the Promotion of Nutritional Therapy
PO Box 47
Heathfield
East Sussex
TN22 8ZX
Tel: +44 143 586 7007

Brazil

João de Deus

www.friendsofthecasa.com
Official website for Joao de Deus. Includes information on etiquette,
protocol of the casa and places to seek accommodation.

Irish company that organises flights to Brazil from Dublin via
Lisbon to Brasilia:

Elliott Travel
Edward Street
Baltinglass
Co. Wicklow
Contact Martina or Fiona on (059) 648 1722

USA

The Brennan School of Healing
PO Box 2005
East Hampton
NY 11937
www.barbarabrennan.com

Donna Eden
Innersource
777E Main Street
Ashland
Oregon 97520
USA
www.innersource.net

Resource Websites

www.wddty.com

www.explorepub.com

www.theragem.com

www.wrf.org

www.toolsforexploration.com

www.tldp.com

www.touch4health.com

www.emofree.com

www.musicacupuncture.com

www.mindlink.co.za

www.acupuncture.com

www.homeopathic.org

www.alternativemedicine.com

Herbal remedies not safe with medication.

RTE website.

Michael MORRISON – 087-2459402.
New Vistas, Limerick – 061-334455.
Hanes Health, Patrick St – 021-4278101.
Caroline O Keeffe, Clonakilty – 086-8270195.

Printed in the United Kingdom by
Lightning Source UK Ltd., Milton Keynes
139740UK00001B/43/P

9 781847 483805

Fatty acid & thyroid liquescence – made in oil
(no carbohydra